M000032497

Handbook of
CLINICAL
CHIROPRACTIC

Lawrence H. Wyatt, DC, DACBR
Chairman
Department of Diagnostic Imaging
Texas Chiropractic College
Pasadena, Texas

AN ASPEN PUBLICATION®
Aspen Publishers, Inc.
Gaithersburg, Maryland
1992

Library of Congress Cataloging-in-Publication Data

Wyatt, Lawrence H.
Handbook of clinical chiropractic /
Lawrence H. Wyatt.
p. cm.
Includes bibliographical references and index.
ISBN: 0-8342-0250-6
1. Chiropractic—Handbooks, manuals, etc. I. Title.
[DNLM: 1. Chiropractic. WB 905 W975h]
RZ242.9.W93 1991
615.5'34—dc20
DNLM/DLC
for Library of Congress
91-22352
CIP

Copyright © 1992 by Aspen Publishers, Inc.
All rights reserved.

Aspen Publishers, Inc., grants permission for photocopying for limited personal
or internal use. This consent does not extend to other kinds of copying, such as
copying for general distribution, for advertising or promotional purposes, for
creating new collective works, or for resale. For information, address
Aspen Publishers, Inc., Permissions Department, 200 Orchard Ridge Drive,
Gaithersburg, Maryland 20878.

The authors have made every effort to ensure the accuracy of the information
herein, particularly with regard to drug selection and dose. However, appropriate
information sources should be consulted, especially for new or unfamiliar drugs or
procedures. It is the responsibility of every practitioner to evaluate the appropri-
ateness of a particular opinion in the context of actual clinical situations and with
due consideration to new developments. Authors, editors, and the publisher cannot
be held responsible for any typographical or other errors found in this book.

Editorial Services: Lisa Hajjar
Daniel N. da Cruz
Library of Congress Catalog Card Number: 91-22352
ISBN: 0-8342-0250-6

Printed in the United States of America

2 3 4 5

To my parents
I love you

Table of Contents

Forewords xi

Preface xv

Acknowledgments xvii

Part I—Record Keeping and Professional
        Protocols 1

Chapter 1—Introduction to Clinical
          Chiropractic 3

        Introduction 3
        Doctor-Patient Relationship 3

Chapter 2—Medical Record Keeping 5

        Introduction 5
        Problem-Oriented Medical
          Record System 6

Chapter 3—Writing Orders 11

        Introduction 11
        Types of Orders 12
        Medication Orders/Prescription
          Writing 13

Chapter 4—Personalized Referral
            Listings   17

        Introduction   17
        When To Refer   17
        Types of Referrals   18

Chapter 5—Hospital Protocols   21

        Introduction   21
        General Hospital Protocols   21

Part II—Clinical Investigation   25

Chapter 6—History and Physical
            Examination   27

        Introduction   27
        Chief Complaint   28
        General History   28
        Physical Examination   32

Chapter 7—Orthopedics   47

        Introduction   47
        Useful Orthopedic Tests   47
        Range of Motion   57
        Scoliosis Evaluation   59
        Spondylolisthesis   62
        Screening Examinations   64

Chapter 8—Neurologic Evaluation   67

        Introduction   67
        Location of the Lesion   67
        Etiology of the Lesion   71
        Treatment of the Lesion
          and Contraindications to
          Treatment   74

Chapter 9—Laboratory Diagnosis   79

        Introduction   79
        Complete Blood Count (CBC) ...   79
        Urinalysis   83
        Serum Chemistries   85
        Special Studies   91
        Special Laboratory Panels   92

Chapter 10—Diagnostic Imaging **95**

    Introduction   95
    Basic Rules of Radiographic
      Interpretation   97
    Differential Diagnosis and
      Follow-Up Imaging   101
    Radiation Physics Made Easy . . .   104

**Chapter 11—Procedures Used in Clinical
         Practice** **113**

    Introduction   113

Part III—Differential Diagnosis **127**

Chapter 12—Rheumatology **129**

    Introduction   129
    Classification of Rheumatologic
      Diseases   129
    History   129
    Physical Examination   131
    Laboratory   132
    Radiology   133
    Rheumatologic Diseases   133

Chapter 13—Clinical Oncology **141**

    Introduction   141
    Screening Methods   141
    Clinical Examination   143
    Laboratory Investigation   146
    Diagnostic Imaging   148

Chapter 14—Spine Pain **151**

    Introduction   151
    Vertebrogenic Spine Pain   151
    Referred Spine Pain   156

Chapter 15—Differential Diagnosis **161**

    Introduction   161
    Abdomen   161
    Chest   165
    Nervous System   168
    Skeleton   173

Chapter 16—Commonly Prescribed
                 Medications with
                 Neuromusculoskeletal Side
                 Effects 175

Part IV—Management Protocols 181

Chapter 17—Sprain/Strain Protocols 183

          Introduction 183
          Bandage/Brace 183
          Rest/Rehabilitation 184
          Apply Ice 185
          Compression 185
          Crutches 185
          Chiropractic Care 186
          Elevation 186
          Unstable Injuries 186

Chapter 18—Cervical Spine Trauma
                 Protocols 189

          Introduction 189
          Examination 189
          Radiography 190
          Physical Therapy 191
          Manipulation 193
          Ancillary Therapies 193

Chapter 19—Low Back Pain Protocols 195

          Introduction 195
          Diagnosis 195
          Treatment 195

Chapter 20—Contraindications to Chiropractic
                 Manipulation 199

          Absolute Contraindications 200
          Relative Contraindications 201

Chapter 21—Physical Therapy in
                 Chiropractic 203

          Introduction 203
          Effects of Physical Therapy
             Modalities 203
          Specific Physical Therapy
             Modalities 203

Chapter 22—Nutrition **213**

    Introduction 213
    General Diet Plans 213
    Nutritional Care for Selected
        Diseases 214

**Appendix A—Abbreviations in
               Chiropractic** **219**

Index **233**

Forewords

One of the greatest rewards a teacher can experience is to see worthwhile achievements from his students. This book by Dr. Wyatt offers such a reward to me. The *Handbook of Clinical Chiropractic* should find wide acceptance by both students and practitioners.

It is concise, to the point, and helpful regarding most areas where doctors of chiropractic may need a quick reference. The bibliographies allow one who has need for greater depth than is offered in the handbook to find such material with ease. One of the strengths of the book is its use of charts and algorithms that not only quickly summarize concepts, but also put them into perspective.

I believe that the book fills a need that is not otherwise met for the practicing chiropractic doctor and the chiropractic student.

Dr. Wyatt's achievements since his residency in radiology at the Los Angeles College of Chiropractic, and this book, which encompasses much more than radiology, show that his energy has not diminished and that he continues his quest for excellence.

Joseph Howe, DC, DACBR
Professor of Radiology
Los Angeles College of Chiropractic
Los Angeles, California

During my 33 years in the field of chiropractic patient care as a practitioner, educator, and lecturer, I have been privileged to observe an astronomical evolution of the profession. The changes have included a broadening of the practice's scope, improving our diagnostic and therapeutic acumen, and ultimately assuming our role in the multidisciplinary arena of patient care.

These changes have opened a dialogue with other allied health care providers to the extent that our skills are accepted and even invited into the numerous versions of hospice care. The field of manipulation has been scientifically proven to be of value in the management of orthopedic patients, and chiropractic has assumed the role of leadership in its application. Such strides have assigned commensurate responsibilities to each and every member of the profession, mandating that each doctor maintain current understanding.

A manual of this type is invaluable in order for our professional colleagues to stay current in the variety of new practice modes in hospitals, rehabilitation facilities, and medico-legal arenas. On a daily basis, each of us finds a need for a quick reference to expedite decisions and judgments in patient management. Dr. Wyatt is to be commended for recognizing the need for such a manual and for persevering to complete it.

John M. Nash, DC, CCSP, FICC
Southwest Diagnostic and Rehabilitation
Houston, Texas
Former Dean of Chiropractic Sciences
Texas Chiropractic College
Pasadena, Texas

I read the *Handbook of Clinical Chiropractic* with great interest. The task of putting together a comprehensive clinical chiropractic handbook is an extraordinary one. Dr. Wyatt has put forth a supreme effort in organizing a succinct and informative manuscript. It was a pleasure reading this text with its easy-to-follow headings and comprehensive evaluations of the various systems in clinical chiropractic diagnosis and treatment. I equate this handbook with the *Merck Manual*, which all of us, as practitioners, have found indispensable over the years. This handbook's chiropractic perspective makes it unique and valuable to the practicing doctor of chiropractic and to the chiropractic student.

The *Handbook of Clinical Chiropractic* is a welcome addition to any chiropractic library and is certainly worthy of purchase by both the chiropractic student and practitioner.

Terry R. Yochum, DC, DACBR
Adjunct Professor of Radiology
Los Angeles College of Chiropractic
Los Angeles, California
Director, Rocky Mountain Chiropractic
Radiological Center
Clinical Instructor of Skeletal Radiology
Department of Radiology
University of Colorado School of Medicine
Denver, Colorado

Preface

This handbook provides the chiropractic student, clerk, intern, and practicing physician with a quick and convenient reference to many of the more common clinical problems unique to the practice of chiropractic.

The coverage of topics in this manual is general, with specific historical, physical, laboratory, imaging, and treatment protocols included where necessary. The reader will find this book filled with lists, algorithms, and other quick-reference material. Should the reader desire a more in-depth understanding of any of the problems in this text, bibliographies are provided.

It is hoped that more accurate diagnoses will emerge with the help of this manual. Best of luck to all.

Acknowledgments

Many hours have been invested in this manuscript but the final product would not have been possible without the help of many people. To all of them I extend my heartfelt thanks and respect for all their efforts. I especially would like to thank "my better half," Cheryl, for her inspiration and encouragement when things looked bleak. She is indeed my best friend. I would also like to thank David Voracek, D.C., for his ideas; T. Sammi Lowe, D.C., for her expertise; and my mentor, Joseph W. Howe, D.C., DACBR, without whom none of my work in chiropractic would have been possible. To Hank Adams, D.C.; Don Boyer, D.C.; Ron Grabowski, D.C., R.D., and T. Sammi Lowe, D.C., go thanks for their contributions to chapters in this text. I would also like to thank Greg Hollier, D.C., and Mike Smith, D.C., for their artistic expertise.

I

Record Keeping and Professional Protocols

1

Introduction to Clinical Chiropractic

INTRODUCTION

Long gone are the days when chiropractic was taught to high school graduates with no college education. The field of chiropractic has rapidly evolved into the second largest branch of health care in the world, and is the largest branch that heals without using drugs. The road has been long and arduous, but the modern chiropractic doctor is now well schooled in the art and science of chiropractic as well as generic medicine. With recent changes in state statutes, many chiropractors are involved in manipulation under anesthesia, minor surgery, analgesia, and use of injectable medications and vitamins. Hospital rotations for chiropractic interns and residents are becoming more popular as well. In light of this rapid metamorphosis, it has become necessary to collate the abundant clinical information applicable to chiropractic practice into an easily understood format. This book was written for that purpose.

DOCTOR-PATIENT RELATIONSHIP

Before addressing the specifics of chiropractic practice, it is appropriate to briefly discuss doctor-patient relationships. The key to gaining and maintaining the trust and compliance of patients is effective interpersonal communication. This can be accomplished in a number of different ways including, but not limited to, the following:

1. Allow the patient to actively participate in the decision-making process as regards a diagnosis and treatment plan.
2. Demonstrate a genuine concern for the patient's feelings and opinions. Too often, doctors fail to realize that the patient will often offer them the diagnosis.
3. Never argue with the patient. Maintaining control over the patient is, without question, necessary; however, the relationship should be cooperative and not adversarial.
4. Solicit the patient's participation in expediting the healing process by having him or her do exercises and other forms of home care. An involved patient is more likely to comply with recommended treatment.
5. Reward the compliant patient.

2

Medical Record Keeping

INTRODUCTION

The "chart" is a record of the patient's health care while under a physician's guidance. It serves as a data base on each and every patient. Statutes require that these records, including radiographs and special studies, be maintained by the physician for a number of years. Many times special requirements concerning the length of time records must be kept on file are made for persons under legal age. All physicians should become familiar with the relevant state statutes where they practice.

Accurate record keeping is essential for chiropractors. Not only will immaculate records assist the physician in collating information concerning the patient, but they will assist the physician if he or she is unfortunately called to court. The patient chart is also helpful when it becomes necessary to produce records for third-party payors. Communication among physicians concerning a patient's status or progress is also notably enhanced with meticulously kept charts.

The patient's chart should be organized so that pertinent information is easily accessible. Disorganization precludes good patient care, as most of the doctor's time is then spent in searching for records instead of on patient management.

A common problem in charting is the misconception that a blank space beside a question or a test is the equivalent of a negative response. A blank space provides the reader with no information whatsoever. All queries and spaces on forms should be answered, thereby leaving no question as to the status of that finding.

Illegible records are also troublesome. Should the patient see another physician, by choice or necessity, legible notes allow the new doctor to interpret the patient's previous health care without delay.

There are a number of useful hints to be used when writing in a patient's chart. Each note should be titled (e.g., "Intern Note") and dated with the time that the patient was seen. The source of the information, especially with pediatric, geriatric, and mentally impaired patients, should be recorded. A signature and title should follow any entry into the records. All charting should be performed on official institutional forms.

So that the medical record does not become a small manuscript ready for publication, only pertinent positives and pertinent negatives should be recorded. Pertinent positives are not difficult to understand. Pertinent negatives should be entered if their inclusion will alter the diagnostic or therapeutic plans for the patient.

PROBLEM-ORIENTED MEDICAL RECORD SYSTEM

There are many different forms of charting, the most popular of which is probably the problem-oriented medical record (POMR) system developed by Dr. Larry Weed. This system permits a standardized analysis of each of the patient's problems with good cross-referencing. The major disadvantage of this system is that it is somewhat more cumbersome than many others.

The POMR system is divided into a number of component parts including the comprehensive data base, problem list, initial plans, and progress notes. Examples of each part can be found in Exhibits 2-1A, 2-1B, and 2-1C.

Comprehensive Data Base

Creation of a problem-oriented medical record begins with the collection of all historical and physical

Exhibit 2-1A Complete Problem List

Complete Problem List

Patient ___JANE DOE___   File number ___1234-56___

Date problem entered	Active	Inactive
4-25-91	X 1. LOW BACK PAIN ──→	DISC BULGE L4/5 (5/2/1991)
	2. RIGHT LEG PAIN ──→	DISC BULGE L4/5 (5/2/1991)
	3.	APPENDICITIS (1973)
	4. DIABETES MELLITUS	
	5.	ENDOMETRIOSIS (1988)
5/4/91	X 6. NECK PAIN	
	X 7. HEADACHE	

Exhibit 2-1B Initial Plans

Initial Plans

Patient ___JANE DOE___   File number ___1234-56___

#1, #2   LOW BACK PAIN; RIGHT LEG PAIN

DX: RULE OUT HERNIATED NUCLEUS PULPOSUS: HISTORY, PHYSICAL, PLAIN FILM LUMBAR SPINE SERIES, MRI LUMBAR SPINE, ___ ___

RULE OUT FACET SYNDROME: HISTORY, PHYSICAL EXAM, PLAIN FILM LUMBAR SPINE SERIES

RULE OUT SPINAL CORD LESION: HISTORY, PHYSICAL EXAM, MRI LUMBAR SPINE, CBC, UA

RX: LUMBAR SPINE MOBILIZATION (GENTLE) UNTIL MRI RESULTS BACK.

PT. EDUC: TOLD HER OF THREE MAIN POSSIBILITIES FOR PAIN AND ADVISED OF DX TESTS WE WILL PERFORM. REST AT HOME. NO HEAVY LIFTING. PERMISSION TO RX OBTAINED WITH INFORMED CONSENT

examination data, supplemented by data from any diagnostic tests that are appropriate for the patient's age, sex, and physical status. Copies of reports of any examinations should become a permanent part of the patient's chart.

Exhibit 2-1C Progress Notes

Progress Notes

Patient: JANE DOE   File number: 1234·56

Date

4-29-91	#1,2 LOW BACK PAIN, RIGHT LEG PAIN
	S: SHE STATES TODAY THAT LEG PAIN IS GONE
	AND LOW BACK PAIN IS ONLY 25% OF ORIGINAL.
	BOWEL/BLADDER FUNCTION INTACT.
	O: STRAIGHT LEG RAISE NEGATIVE TO 90° FULL
	RANGE OF MOTION WITH MILD PAIN DURING
	EXTENSION. DEEP TENDON REFLEXES INTACT
	NO PARESTHESIA. L4/5 FIXED IN LEFT ROTATION.
	A: FACET SYNDROME L4/5. RESOLVING WELL.
	P: DX: MRI RESULTS = WITHIN NORMAL LIMITS.
	RX: FLEXION DISTRACTION X 10 MOTIONS.
	ALTERNATING KNEE-TO-CHEST EXERCISES.
	PT. EDUC: ADVISED HER SHE IS PROGRESSING
	WELL. WILL REDUCE RX TO 1 X/WK AND
	RE-EXAMINE ON 5-1-91.

Problem List

The problem list is a compilation of the patient's problems, both past and present, often collected from the comprehensive data base. Each problem is recorded and dated in descending order of severity on a problem list sheet and assigned a number for future reference. Patient problems can be a symptom, sign, abnormal laboratory finding, abnormal diagnostic imaging study, or abnormal special study. The problem that has brought the patient to the physician's attention is marked with an asterisk to identify it as the chief complaint. Each problem is also listed as active (still causing the patient distress) or inactive (no longer a problem for the patient). Inactive problems are listed with the date they became inactive. As the signs, symptoms, and other problems are collated to form a specific diagnosis, the problem list should be updated accordingly by deleting the compilation of problems previously noted and noting a diagnosis as a new active problem.

Initial Plans

The initial plans list the diagnostic and therapeutic procedures to be performed on the patient, along with their rationale, as well as patient education plans.

Initial plans should be formulated for any active problem on the problem list. This rule applies even if the problem is not treatable with chiropractic health care, in which case a note stating that the problem is being handled by another physician will suffice. If the problem is to be comanaged, that fact should also be noted.

Listing the rationale for procedures is important, as it forces the doctor to justify the necessity of the test or therapy to be performed. Any diagnostic test required should contribute significant data to the diagnosis or prognosis for the patient. There are also admission protocols, which vary with each institution, that are many times performed. For example, any patient with an acute cervical acceleration-deceleration injury (whiplash) may be required to have a Davis series of radiographs performed while in a cervical collar. Complete blood count and urinalysis are often part of an admission protocol as well.

Progress Notes

Progress notes are a short notation of the progress or regress in the patient's status. Each active problem being treated by the doctor, with its appropriate number from the problem list, should be recorded. There are four divisions of the progress notes, which form the mnemonic SOAP.

- *Subjective*—New symptoms or a change in symptoms since the last note. These are expressed in the patient's words, if that format is appropriate. Have the patient quantify the symptoms, if at all possible. For example, if the patient had one dollar's worth of pain on the first visit, have him or her quantify how much pain is still being experienced—e.g., 50 cents worth of pain.

- *Objective*—New or changed examination, laboratory, or imaging findings since the last note. Again, quantify the changes if possible. For example, a straight leg test that was initially positive at 45 degrees and now is not positive until 75 degrees helps quantify the amount of patient progress.

- *Assessment*—Diagnosis(es), whether working or final, along with any concomitant and complicating factors. These should be as specific as possible.

- *Plans*—New or continuing diagnostic, therapeutic, or patient education plans. For example, if it is important that the patient remain in bed for three days with only bathroom privileges until the results of a computerized tomography scan are known, this should be noted. Specific types of manipulation, physical therapy, or any other therapeutic procedure; their location; and the patient's tolerance of any procedures performed should also be charted.

Specialized Notes

Many institutions will add an admission note and a discharge note. These notes summarize the patient's status at admission to the facility and at the time of discharge from care, including the patient's complaint, status, and progress. For discharge notes, the reason for discharge should also be noted. If the patient is discharged after not following a diagnostic or treatment plan, then a "discharged against medical advice" form should be signed by the patient. It is important for medicolegal reasons to inform the patient of the reason for the discharge. In cases of discharge against medical advice, it is vital to suggest another doctor and emphasize the importance of the patient seeking further care.

Informed consent should be obtained from patients undergoing diagnostic and therapeutic procedures. A witness should also sign the informed consent form. In the case of a minor, parental or guardian consent is also necessary.

Operative notes may be used in some instances. Patients undergoing manipulation under anesthesia or conscious sedation will also require a specialized note.

BIBLIOGRAPHY

Larson, E.B., and M.S. Eisenberg. 1987. *Manual of admitting orders and therapeutics.* Philadelphia: Harcourt Brace Jovanovich.

Mootz, R. 1988. Chiropractic clinical management and record keeping. *International Review of Chiropractic.* 44(3):56–61.

Walker, H.K. 1980. *Clinical methods: The history, physical and laboratory examinations.* Boston: Butterworth Publishers, Inc.

3

Writing Orders

INTRODUCTION

Orders are instructions to patients, assistants, interns, clerks, and consultants concerning the management of a case. They can be general or specific depending upon what is required. For example, an order for "Vitamin C as needed (prn) for acute coryza" is obviously inadequate because no dosage or route of administration is noted. A complete order should state the order, date, and time; what is to be administered; to whom, how, and when it is to be given; and where it is to be administered.

There are many templates for writing orders. *Standing orders* (SO) are instructions that are to be performed on specific types of patients under specific circumstances without the need for consultation with the clinician. For example, if a patient has been involved in a motor vehicle accident, the SO might be for a seven-view cervical spine (Davis) series, the lateral being performed while the patient is in a cervical collar.

Orders that vary and require discussion with the attending clinician before being performed may be given by the clinician as *written orders* (WO), *verbal orders* (VO), or *telephone orders* (TO). The type of orders given should be placed in the patient's chart next to the orders.

If the words *STAT* or *ASAP* appear next to a set of orders they should be performed immediately and supersede any routine investigations being performed.

Of course, all chart entries require the signature of a licensed doctor.

Orders are the backbone of chiropractic diagnosis and therapy. The more concise and easily understood the orders, the better those interacting on a particular case, including the patient, can effectively carry out those orders.

TYPES OF ORDERS

The orders described in this chapter can be easily remembered by the mnemonic LATER DUDES, (representing laboratory, activity, treatment, extras, radiology and diagnosis, updates, disability, exercises, and supplements). Each element is briefly described below.

- *Laboratory*—Many facilities have admission protocols concerning laboratory studies. Other studies specific to the case at hand should also be noted. All laboratory orders should include when the studies are to be performed and who the ordering doctor is.

- *Activity*—Due to the unique nature of patients seen by chiropractic physicians, all patients should be required to adhere to the level of activity (both work and leisure) prescribed for them. Terms such as light and regular work duty can be used but should be modified by noting both included and excluded activities (e.g., no lifting involving any low back torque). If the patient's activity is unrestricted, the phrase "activities of daily living as much as wanted" (ADL ad. lib.) can be used.

- *Treatment*—The type of treatment, including adjustment and manipulation, physical therapy, medication, rehabilitation, and patient instructions should be outlined. Be as specific as possible, including frequency, duration, and dosage where applicable. Manipulation should be ordered prn (pro re nata, or "as needed"). The type and location of the manipulation should be charted as specifically as possible in the progress notes. Contraindications for any type of procedure should be listed here as well.

- *Extras*—This is where orders for any special diagnostic studies, such as an electromyogram (EMG), or special treatment or consultations, such as "neurosurgical consultation to rule out (R/O) cord tumor," should be made. Any special requirements for preparation for these tests should be given to the patient and duly noted. Any orders that do not fit into any of the other categories should be included here.

- *Radiology*—Any requisitions for diagnostic radiography should be included here. Be as specific as possible concerning which views are to be performed and any special preparatory procedures (e.g., cleansing enema) of which the patient should be aware.
- *Diagnosis*—The working clinical diagnosis, including pertinent rule outs, should be included here.
- *Updates*—Reexamination dates and dates for follow-up x-ray, laboratory, and special studies are explained here. The specific examinations and tests to be performed should be listed.
- *Disability*—The amount of disability suffered by the patient should be noted here. The percentage of disability according to standard disability evaluation procedures should be recorded also, if applicable. Any home care instructions for the patient, either by the patient or patient's family, are noted.
- *Exercises*—The type and frequency of exercises to be performed by the patient and the instructions given to the patient should be charted. Specific weights to be used during exercises must be noted.
- *Supplements*—Any nutritional supplementation, including dosage, route of administration, and frequency, should be noted. If written instructions for the patient were given, they should be recorded in the chart.

Using this form of order writing will assure the doctor of excellent patient care and compliance, as the orders can be understood and carried out precisely.

MEDICATION ORDERS/PRESCRIPTION WRITING

Although prescription writing for medications does not occur often in the chiropractic profession, there are states that do allow such prescribing privileges. The following is a format for proper prescription writing (see also Exhibit 3-1). This format may be used for medications, physical therapy, supplements, orthopedic supports, and other such necessities.

Essential components of a prescription include:

- *Name, age, and address.*
- *Date*—State regulations vary but most states require that a prescription be filled within six months. Check with your state for specific requirements.
- *Rx*—Rx is from the Latin for "recipe." The product or therapy being prescribed and its strength and type (generic or brand name) should be noted. The form of the product (e.g., tablets, capsules) should also be included.
- *Dispense ("disp")*—The amount (e.g., number of tablets) or the time period (e.g., six weeks) for the treatment is noted here.
- *Sig*—Sig is from the Latin "signa," which means "mark through." This is where the patient instructions are noted. This portion of the prescription is typically written in shorthand. (Abbreviations are listed in Appendix A.)
- *Refills*—This lists the number of times the prescription can be filled.

Exhibit 3-1 Typical Prescription Form

```
+--------------------------------------------------+
|             John Q. Public, D.C.                 |
|               123 Anywhere Street                |
|              Anyplace, Texas 55555               |
|--------------------------------------------------|
| Name: _____  Age: ____   |
| Address: _____  Date: ____  |
|--------------------------------------------------|
| Rx:                                              |
|                                                  |
|    Ibuprofen                     200 mg          |
|       disp. #25 tablets                          |
|                                                  |
|    Sig: Take three tablets three times per day as|
|         needed for pain.                         |
|                                                  |
| Doctor: _____         |
+--------------------------------------------------+
```

Prescriptions should be written on a prescription pad containing the doctor's name, address, license number, and Drug Enforcement Administration number (when applicable). There should also be a place for the physician's signature. All notations should be printed and clearly legible.

If instructions to patients are given, they should not be abbreviated or written in shorthand. Instead, they should be written out and easily understood.

BIBLIOGRAPHY

Berkow, Robert, ed. 1982. *The Merck manual of diagnosis and therapy*. 14th ed. Rahway, N.J.: Merck Sharp & Dohme Laboratories.

Dornbrand, L., A. Hoole, R. Fletcher, and G. Pickard, eds. 1985. *Manual of clinical problems in adult ambulatory care*. Boston: Little, Brown & Co.

Larson, E.B., and M.S. Eisenberg. 1987. *Manual of admitting orders and therapeutics*. Philadelphia: Harcourt Brace Jovanovich.

4

Personalized Referral Listings

INTRODUCTION

The referral of a patient for further diagnosis or therapeutic care is at times helpful and many times a necessity. Referrals may be within the chiropractic profession or to some other branch of health care.

With the improvements in communication, technology, and education made during the last decade, health care professionals are forming relationships thought in the past to be improbable, if not impossible. Today's chiropractor must understand how, when, why, and where to refer a patient. To converse with other disciplines about patients, it is necessary to be fluent in spinal- and biomechanical-related disorders as well as general health care.

An important point to bear in mind is that quality referrals foster rapport and cross-referrals among physicians.

WHEN TO REFER

When a patient fails to respond to chiropractic care or reaches a point where further improvement is unlikely from spinal manipulation and other forms of therapy, referral becomes necessary. It is of extreme importance that clinical data obtained from the patient's history, physical, and special examinations, along with treatment and response to therapy, be well documented. These data provide an accurate reflec-

17

tion of the patient's progress, or lack thereof. Only at this point can an intelligent decision regarding referral be made.

Referral is also necessary when a patient presents with a disorder whose treatment is outside the scope of chiropractic. Examples might include patients with cancer, active heart disease, prestroke syndromes, abdominal aortic aneurysms, and diabetes mellitus.

TYPES OF REFERRALS

There are two directions of referral: from the chiropractic office to another physician, or vice versa. Protocols will differ depending on the direction of the referral.

Referral to Another Physician

Exhibit 4-1 contains a summary of guidelines for referring to another physician. Before making a referral, the chiropractor should discuss with the patient the need for further services and answer any questions he or she may have; contact the appropriate specialist's office to arrange an appointment (speaking directly to the physician if necessary); and compose a report that includes the following vital information:

- History
- Family history
- Physical examination findings
- Special examination findings
- Therapeutic procedures already utilized

Exhibit 4-1 Outgoing Referral Guidelines

Discuss need for services with patient.
Contact appropriate consultant.
Schedule appointment.
Send referral report.
Follow up with consultant.

The referral should state any requirements regarding disposition of the case as one of the following: diagnosis only, diagnosis and treatment of this condition only, or diagnosis and treatment of this and future conditions. All requests should be as specific as possible. A brief, concise and clearly written consultation/referral request letter is a must. It is imperative that the referring physician fully communicate the nature of the problem. A communication breakdown only detracts from good patient care and many times alienates the patient, who is subject to conflicting opinions from various doctors.

If the referring physician wishes to be present at any procedures performed on the patient, including surgery, that request should be included in the consultation request.

It is the responsibility of the primary physician to coordinate the patient's care. It is paramount that no clinician demean another in front of the patient. Disagreements do and will continue to occur. These are disputes between physicians and should not be brought to the patient's attention.

Finally, the referring physician should request either a verbal report, written report, or both from the specialist.

Referrals from Another Physician

The other direction of referral is an incoming patient from some other physician. The referring physician now requires a thorough, complete, and timely report from the receiving physician with his or her recommendations. A brief thank you for the referral and confirmation of the patient's appointment date and time should also be provided.

The receiving physician's responsibilities when receiving a patient from another health care professional vary according to the nature of the referral (see Exhibit 4-2). It is important to ascertain the exact nature of the consultation from the referring doctor so that the proper examination and/or treatment may be accomplished. Results of consultations with the patient, history of the patient, and a physical examination of the areas in question and any important ancillary examinations are always necessary for the protection of the doctor accepting the referral. Special examinations include imaging and laboratory investi-

Exhibit 4-2 Incoming Referral Guidelines

Ascertain reason for referral.
Consult with patient.
Review history and perform a physical examination.
Perform any special examinations.
Supply a written report of findings, treatment, and
recommendations.

---

gations, diagnostic impressions, including a written
report; treatment recommendations; and treatment
when requested. It is also vital to ascertain if the referring doctor wishes to be present during the examina-
tion(s) and/or treatment.

Communication is the key to any referral. The more
accurately the proper protocols are followed, the more
the patient benefits and the better the interprofes-
sional relationships among doctors become. Every
doctor should keep a referral list with relevant information about specialists in the area (see Exhibit 4-3).

Exhibit 4-3 Personalized Referral List

Doctor's Name	Telephone	Speciality

5

Hospital Protocols

INTRODUCTION

With the advent of medical and surgical rotations for interns and hospital admitting privileges for chiropractic doctors, it has become necessary for clinicians to become familiar with hospital protocols. Knowledge of the proper procedures used in the hospital setting will allow for rapid integration into the hospital system.

GENERAL HOSPITAL PROTOCOLS

As a general rule, the expectations of an intern on rotation will be explained at the outset. It is imperative that one understand these responsibilities and protocols and become familiar with schedules for operating suites, rounds, clinics, and conferences. Punctuality is essential since hospitals generally operate on a very tight schedule.

In order to save time, one should be aware of the location of each of the various departments in the hospital. Introducing oneself to clerks and secretaries can also be useful, as can carrying a small book with room locations, telephone numbers, names, and a daily schedule.

Case Presentations

There are generally two types of case presentations: formal and informal. Keeping notes on an index card on the patient being presented is very useful.

Informal presentations are usually given to small groups and consist of a pertinent and concise report of history, examination findings, and treatments administered to patients since their admission. These are typically from one to five minutes in length. Formal presentations, on the other hand, are usually presented to larger groups, typically at a conference. These presentations cover the patient's entire medical history and are usually from ten to twenty minutes in length. Interns should check with the chief of the service for exact instructions regarding presentations. In any event, the presenting intern should know the patient as well as possible.

Charting Procedures

Although the problem-oriented medical record keeping system is outlined in this text and is commonly used, it is not the system used in all hospitals. The chiropractic physician should become familiar with whatever system is used in the hospital.

Clinics and Ward Rounds

It is necessary that physicians become familiar with history and physical examination procedures commonly used in the hospital. Imaging studies and protocols also vary between institutions. Finally, it is expected that interns on rotation, especially in internal and family medicine services, will become somewhat knowledgeable regarding drugs of choice for the diseases most commonly seen in each respective facility.

Surgery

Learning the surgical procedures in an operating room (OR) can make one's observation much more meaningful and worthwhile. The surgical suite can be one of the most instructional experiences of a career.

It is absolutely necessary that sterile technique be used in the OR. Preparations for surgery involve the following:

- Don a pair of surgical scrubs after all clothing is removed (including T-shirts). Tuck the scrub top into the bottoms.
- Move from the locker room and obtain a mask, cap, and shoe covers. Men with beards should wear full caps. All hair must be covered.
- Before scrubbing, remove all jewelry and nail polish and put on the surgical mask when close to the scrub sinks. (A mask must be worn in all areas except the OR hallways, unless near the scrub sinks in the hallways.)
- If contamination occurs during scrubbing, begin the entire procedure over again. (The purpose of scrubbing is to remove bacteria from the skin of the hands and arms.) Check with the surgeon before deviating from standard scrubbing protocols.
- After completing the hand scrub, back into the OR and dry hands. Always keep hands above elbows until fully gowned and gloved.
- After drying, hold arms out straight in front and allow a nurse to slip on the gown. Another nurse will tie the back string (remember, one's back is not sterile). The nurse will then hold out a surgical glove. Push hands through the gloves. Make sure the gloves are free of any holes. Double gloving may be necessary in patients with highly contagious diseases, such as AIDS and hepatitis. Finish this procedure by giving the front string of the gown to the nurse, turn in place, and then tie the strings together. The surgeon may now instruct that the powder be wiped off the gloves.
- After being fully scrubbed, gowned, and gloved, ascertain where one should be located and stand there with hands above waist in the praying position. Do not cross arms.
- If the surgeon makes a request, perform it precisely while remaining sterile. When moving around the OR, pass sterile areas with the front of the body and nonsterile areas with the back.
- If someone in the OR says you have been contaminated, accept that fact and do what is deemed necessary to assure your sterility.
- When unscrubbed or nonsterile in the OR, remain at least one foot from any sterile areas and do not touch anything that is sterile.

II

Clinical Investigation

6

History and Physical Examination

INTRODUCTION

The history is the first step in the evaluation of any patient's chief complaint. It has been said many times that a good clinical history almost always will lead the physician to the correct diagnosis. It is for this reason that this chapter emphasizes obtaining an adequate clinical history.

The first step in taking a history is to be a good listener. Too often the diagnosis is lost because the physician fails to let the patient adequately explain the signs and symptoms he or she is experiencing.

Another helpful hint is to ask the patient open-ended questions rather than questions that suggest the response being sought from the patient. For example, it is better to ask "Are you experiencing any pain anywhere else?" than "You aren't experiencing any pain in your legs, are you?" The latter suggests to the patient that a negative answer is expected. Questions should be phrased in terms that the patient fully understands; medical terminology should be avoided. "Are you experiencing any pain below your breastbone?" is better than "Are you experiencing any substernal angina?"

It is also important to remember to record a negative response from a patient as "the patient denies leg pain" rather than "the patient has not had any leg pain." This will help to protect the physician if the case is called to court.

CHIEF COMPLAINT

The chief complaint is the reason for the patient's visit and is recorded in the patient's own words. It may become obvious later during examination that this complaint is not the patient's most serious problem, but it is the starting point of all good clinical workups.

A number of factors concerning the chief complaint must be obtained. These are included in the mnemonic OPPQRST and represent the events of the present illness.

- *Onset*—When did this complaint begin?
- *Provocative factors*—What worsens the complaint?
- *Palliative factors*—What relieves the complaint?
- *Quality*—What type of pain is it?
- *Radiation*—Does the pain radiate to other areas of the body?
- *Setting*—When does the complaint occur?
- *Timing*—How long does the complaint last?

As the patient answers these questions, it will become obvious that other follow-up questions are necessary to help the clinician collate all the information pertinent to the history of the present illness (HPI). Any dates and times included in the HPI should be accurate. Follow-up questions are helpful in confirming or denying what the patient has already said. After the follow-up questioning, the clinician may wish to repeat the HPI back to the patient for further confirmation.

GENERAL HISTORY

In taking the general history, the following components, represented by the mnemonic AMPLE, are reviewed.

Allergies

The presence of allergies to drugs, foods, and other substances should be noted. If the patient denies any allergies, the acronym for no known drug allergies, NKDA, can be used. If there is reason to suspect that the physician will prescribe medication, specific questions regarding that agent and any like it are in order.

Medications

Any medications the patient is currently taking, including analgesics and oral contraceptive agents, should be noted. The dosage, route of administration, and intended purpose of the drug(s) should also be charted. Any adverse reactions should be noted, with the type and severity of the reaction.

Past Medical History (PMH)

The mnemonic HISTORY is used in remembering the physical elements of the PMH.

- *Hospitalizations*—a chronological record of the patient's hospitalizations, with the reason for admission, treatment, and any complications
- *Injuries*—any trauma the patient has sustained, including date of trauma, treatment, and outcome for each event
- *Sugar Diabetes*—family or patient history of diabetes mellitus or any other diseases such as myocardial infarction, cerebrovascular accident, or liver, kidney, or lung disease, including dates, treatments, and any sequelae
- *Tumors*—any history of cancer, including type of cancer, date of diagnosis, treatment, and outcome
- *Operations*—any surgical procedures, especially those related to the chief complaint, including date of and reason for surgery as well as clinical outcome and complications
- *Review of Systems (ROS)*—the review of each of the organ systems of the body (see Table 6-1)
- *Youth Diseases*—childhood diseases and immunizations; important, as may offer the final clue to an elusive diagnosis

Family History

A record of relatives' health, including causes of death and ages at time of death of deceased family

Table 6-1 Elements in the Review of Systems (ROS)

System	Symptom
General	Weight change, fatigue, anorexia, weakness, fever, chills, changes in activity
Skin	Rashes, eruptions, changes in warts or moles, pigmentation changes, bruising, itching, hair loss, nail changes
Head	Trauma, headaches, dizziness, lightheadedness
Eyes	Change in acuity of vision, use of corrective lenses, loss of vision, diplopia, photophobia, blurred vision, scotomata, pain, excessive lacrimation, redness, discharge
Ears	Changes in hearing, deafness, tinnitus, discharge, pain, vertigo, otitis
Nose	Rhinorrhea, epistaxis, allergies, airway obstruction
Mouth and throat	Ulcers, tooth pain/extractions, temporomandibular joint (TMJ) pain, gum bleeding, soreness, swelling, enlarged glands, sore throat, strep throat
Neck	Stiffness, lumps/swelling/masses, pain
Lungs	Cough (productive/nonproductive), hemoptysis, dyspnea, pain with respiration, wheezing, night sweats
Cardiac	Palpitations, chest pain, orthopnea, paroxysmal nocturnal dyspnea, ankle swelling, syncope
Vascular	Raynaud's phenomenon, intermittent claudication, hypertension, rheumatic fever
Breasts	Self-examination frequency/results, pain, nipple discharge, lumps/masses, skin dimpling
Gastrointestinal	Usual diet, dysphagia, regurgitation, dyspepsia, nausea, vomiting, belching, abdominal pain, cramps, hematemesis, stool color changes, diarrhea, constipation, change in bowel habits, jaundice, abdominal swelling
Genitourinary	Polyuria, nocturia, oliguria, dysuria, urgency, incontinence, urine color changes, hematuria, sexually transmitted diseases, dyspareunia, scrotal mass (male), hernia
Endocrine	Polydypsia, polyphagia, temperature intolerance, tremors, goiter, alopecia, hirsutism, menstruation history, pregnancy history, dysmenorrhea, premenstrual syndrome, climacteric
Hematopoietic	Anemia, abnormal bleeding, lymph node enlargement/pain
Musculoskeletal	Bone/joint pain, swelling, joint deformity, trauma, restricted range of motion, weakness, atrophy
Neurological	Cranial nerve deficits, seizures, loss of consciousness, paralysis, tremors, ataxia, loss of balance, numbness, paresthesias
Psychologial	Mood swings, depression, anxiety, phobias

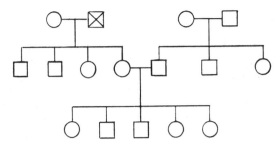

Note: □ = male; ○ = female; X = dead (cause of death and disease for each individual should be noted).

Figure 6-1 Family History Tree

members (Figure 6-1 illustrates a typical family history tree.).

Psychosocial History

Queries regarding home and sex life as well as the patient's normal activities of daily living (ADL), especially with regard to how present complaint may be interfering with any of those activities. Alcohol and drug use should also be documented. Cigarette smoking should be charted as the number of packs per day multiplied by the number of years smoking. The result will be a number of "pack years." This value better serves the clinician in that it better represents the amount the patient has smoked.

Last Menstrual Period

The day of onset of the last menstrual period is important for both the history and the assessment of the ability to x-ray the patient. This is explained in the chapter on diagnostic imaging.

Events of the Present Illness

The characteristics of the present illness are assessed by asking the patient a number of questions. These questions are outlined in the section in this chapter on chief complaint.

PHYSICAL EXAMINATION

The complement to the clinical history is the physical examination, an art that has been forsaken by many and replaced by advanced diagnostic testing. It is unfortunate that procedures that for so many years helped clinicians arrive at a diagnosis have been replaced by testing that is most times expensive and many times unnecessary. Most often the proper diagnosis can be ascertained from a good history and physical examination.

Physical examination skills are learned only through repetition. The more normal findings are seen, felt, and heard, the easier the task of ascertaining the abnormalities common to clinical practice becomes.

General Signs

The physical examination should begin as soon as the clinician sees the patient, with an overview of the bodily habitus and general health. The amount of distress displayed by the patient, such as through facial grimacing, a limp, or protection of the affected part, should be noted. Also, whether a patient's stated age is in concert with his or her apparent age should be determined.

The patient's affect (i.e., overall emotional state) can be assessed by simply conversing with the patient and noting his or her alertness and orientation to time, place, identity, and the present situation.

Vital Signs

Record data on the following vital bodily functions.

- Temperature (oral, rectal, or axillary)
- Pulse rate (with regularity of rate and rhythm)
- Respiratory rate
- Blood pressure (supine, seated, and standing, if necessary)

Hints

- Normal oral temperature varies diurnally between 96.5°F (35.9°C) and 99.1°F (37.3°C);

hence a patient may have a body temperature below 98.6°F and still have a low-grade fever.

- A patient who is febrile has an infection until proven otherwise.
- Respirations are counted after the pulse is noted but before the clinician's hand is removed from the patient's wrist to prevent the patient from voluntarily changing his or her respiratory rate.
- The diagnosis of hypertension (>140/90) requires three separate measurements at least six hours apart.

Skin

The temperature, color, and consistency of the skin along with the presence of any scars, tattoos, moles, unusual hair distribution, or rashes are noted. The presence of itching and tenderness are important signs for differential diagnosis.

Hints

- Cyanosis presents as blue discoloration of the skin.
- Jaundiced patients have a yellowing of the skin and sclera.
- Malignant skin lesions are typically painless. Any mole that changes in size, shape, or consistency is malignant until proven otherwise.

Head/Face

Examination of the head includes assessment of size and shape along with hair distribution and any visible skin lesions. Tender areas are also noted. The presence of any facial deformities suggestive of certain diseases is recorded.

Hints

- The bruits of intracranial tumors, aneurysms, and arteriovenous malformations can be auscultated with the bell of the stethoscope.

- Hypothyroid patients present with a "moon facies" and acromegalics have prognathism, a protruding mandible.

Eyes

The eyes should be examined for any of the following:

- *Eyelids*—Inability to close the lids, edema, drooping (ptosis), and the presence of entropion or extropion.
- *Lacrimal Apparatus*—Overflowing tears (epiphora) and blockage of the nasolacrimal duct, palpation of the lacrimal gland for size and tenderness.
- *Conjunctiva/Sclera*—Unusual scleral color and the presence of nodules. Is there any redness of the conjunctiva? The lower lid should be everted and the "redness" of the internal aspect of the lid estimated.
- *Pupil/Iris*—Unusual size or shape of the pupil and iris along with defects in the iris. Pupillary reflex is challenged for direct and consensual response. Any asymmetry in pupillary size is also noted.
- *Extraocular Muscles*—The six cardinal positions of gaze (Figure 6-2); any nystagmus and its characteristics, any deviation of the eyes (strabismus). The motions of the eyes and their respective cranial nerve supply are represented by the formula

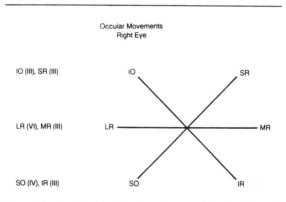

Figure 6-2 Cardinal Positions of Gaze and Ocular Muscle Movement

LR6 SO4 A03 (lateral rectus/CN VI, superior oblique/CN IV, all others/CN III).

- *Visual Acuity*—Acuity checked with Snellen chart. Note if the vision was checked with corrective lenses.
- *Visual Fields*—Fields checked by the confrontation method. A general estimation of the size of each field is made.
- *Ocular Pressure*—A general estimation of pressure, made by palpating the globe. Any right-to-left asymmetry is noted.
- *Fundoscopic Examination*—Any defects in the red reflex (cataracts) and their position and shape. Are there any abnormalities of the retina, optic disc, macula, or microvasculature?

Hints

- Yellow sclera is consistent with jaundice. Blue sclera is found with osteogenesis imperfecta.
- Pallor of the internal aspects of the lower lids is consistent with anemia.
- An Argyll Robertson pupil (syphilis) is one that is small and responds to accommodation but not to light.
- Unequal pupil size in geriatric patients (anisocoria) is not uncommon.
- Paralysis or palsy of an extraocular muscle should lead to a search for intracranial pathology as the primary concern.
- A swollen optic disc (papilledema) suggests an increase in intracranial pressure.
- Loss of temporal vision bilaterally (bitemporal hemianopia) is consistent with a sellar or suprasellar lesion.

Ears

External Examination

Examination of the ears begins with inspection of the pinna, tragus, and antitragus for any visible lesions. A slight tug should be placed on the outer ear and any pain and its location noted. The presence and type of discharge from the external auditory canal is also important.

Otoscopic Examination

Any wax buildup and lesions in the external canal are visually examined. The tympanic membrane is checked for normal light reflex, any defects, fluid behind the membrane, and infection of the membrane itself.

Auditory Examination

Weber's test, the Rinne test, watch ticking, and finger rubbing are ways to check hearing. If impairment is found, audiometry is indicated to define the loss as sensorineural or conductive in nature.

Hints

- Chalky white deposits in the pinna are classically associated with gout.
- A blue-black discoloration of the external ear is found in alkaptonuria (ochronosis).
- Pain with movement of the pinna is consistent with otitis externa (swimmer's ear).
- The external auditory canal is a relatively common location for psoriasis.
- The most common cause of hearing loss is cerumen (wax) buildup in the external canal.

Nose

The normal midline position of the septum is checked, as is the presence of any discharge. Speculum examination includes checks for obstruction, lesions, mucosal color, and tenderness. Finally, sinusitis may be revealed by tapping on the skin over each of the sinuses. The sinuses may then be trans-illuminated for detection of fluid.

Hints

The most common cause of nosebleeds (epistaxis) is nose picking. A pale, bluish discoloration of the nasal mucosa is indicative of hay fever (allergic rhinitis).

Throat

The teeth, lips, and gums are assessed for lesions that can signal systemic illness. The oropharynx is inspected for redness, lesions, and tonsillar swelling (if the tonsils are present). The gag reflex is also tested with a tongue depressor. Ask the patient to stick out his or her tongue to test the integrity of cranial nerve XII.

Hints

- Oral candidiasis is classically associated with diabetes mellitus and acquired immunodeficiency syndrome (AIDS).
- Leukoplakia is considered a precancerous lesion.
- The uvula deviates to the unaffected side with cranial nerve X lesions. The tongue deviates to the affected side with cranial nerve XII lesions.

Thorax

Inspection

Asymmetry and abnormal shapes are noted as well as unilateral inspiratory insufficiency. The respiratory rate is noted (normal = 12–18/minute). Any labored breathing is also recorded.

Palpation

Chest expansion (normal = 2.5–5.0 cm) and any paradoxical motion suggestive of a flail chest should be charted. Is there any palpable tenderness or deformity?

Percussion

Checks for normal diaphragmatic excursion (2–5 cm) and tactile fremitus are performed. Percussion in each of intercostal spaces is also made and the type of percussion note charted.

Auscultation

Begin with the posterior chest and listen in a systematic manner comparing right to left for asymmetry, and finish with the anterior chest. Note any adventitious sounds such as rales, rhonchi, and wheezes. Also listen for an increase in the expiratory phase of respiration suggestive of chronic obstructive pulmonary disease. If indicated, perform egophony, whispered pectoriloquy, and bronchophony tests.

Hints

- Use the bell of the stethoscope to auscultate to lung apices and the diaphragm for the remainder of the examination.
- Emphysema patients are acyanotic and tachypneic (pink puffers) and have a barrel-shaped chest.
- Congestive heart failure patients may demonstrate Cheyne-Stokes respiration (see Figure 6-3).

Heart

Peripheral Examination

The cardiovascular examination begins with a check for cyanosis and clubbing of the digits. The radial and carotid pulses are then palpated for rate, rhythm, and character, and the blood pressure is checked. The remainder of the peripheral pulses are then checked.

Inspection

The precordium is inspected for any abnormal bulges or pulsations and also for the position of the apical impulse. If indicated, the jugular venous pulse is examined in the patient's neck by noting the height of the pulse above the level of the sternal notch.

Palpation

Palpation is used to confirm inspection findings, find any thrills ("palpable murmur"), and locate the point of maximum intensity of the apical impulse. It is usually found in the fifth intercostal space in the midclavicular line in the left hemithorax.

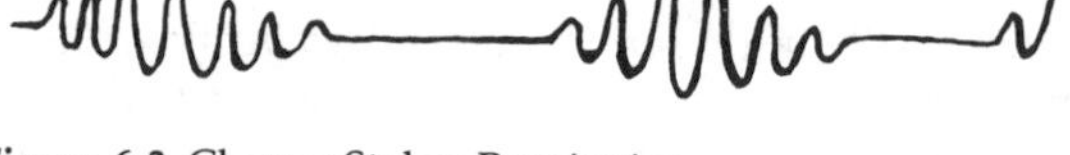

Figure 6-3 Cheyne-Stokes Respiration

Percussion

Percussion of the heart is usually deferred but can be used to outline its borders.

Auscultation

Each of the five auscultatory areas (Figure 6-4) are examined. The heart sounds (S_1,S_2), systole, diastole, and any adventitious sounds, such as pericardial friction rubs, are identified. Murmurs should be classified as to coarse and fine, timing, quality, intensity, and area of maximum intensity and radiation. Special maneuvers may also be used to accentuate murmurs. Figure 6-5 outlines the more common cardiac murmurs and Table 6-2 describes the grading system for murmurs.

Hints

- Listen to the heart with both diaphragm and bell, as low pitch sounds are best heard with the bell and high pitch sounds with the diaphragm.
- A split of the S_1 heart sound is usually of no clinical concern.

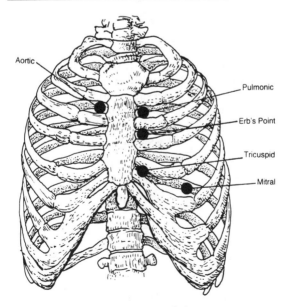

Figure 6-4 Areas for Cardiac Ausculation

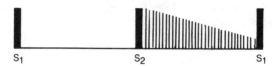

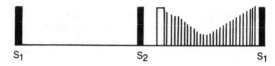

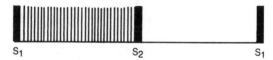

Figure 6-5 Common Cardiac Murmurs

- A third heart sound (S_3) may be normal, but a fourth sound (S_4) is considered pathologic, usually indicating congestive heart failure. S_3 is heard in early diastole while S_4 is heard in late diastole.
- Systolic murmurs are often physiologic in young thin patients. A diastolic murmur should **never** be considered normal.

Table 6-2 Murmur Grading System

Grade	Explanation
1	Barely audible
2	Soft but distinctly audible
3	Loud but no thrill
4	Loud with thrill
5	Loud with palpable thrill
6	Heard with stethoscope off chest

- The normal JVP is <5 cm above the sternal notch. An elevated pressure is consistent with right heart failure.
- Left heart failure causes pulmonary signs and right heart failure causes peripheral signs.
- Pressure on the liver while the patient lies supine can produce an increase in the visible jugular pulse (hepatojugular reflux).

Abdomen

Inspection

The shape and size of the abdomen and umbilicus, and the presence of any dilated veins, skin lesions, scars, and striae are noted. A check should also be made for any visible peristalsis, abnormal pulsations, and distension.

Auscultation

All four quadrants of the abdomen are auscultated for bowel sound quantity (normal = 3–30/minute) and quality. The regions of abdominal vasculature should be checked for the presence of bruits, which are consistent with abnormal flow from atherosclerosis or aneurysm. Figure 6-6 graphically displays the normal position of abdominal vessels.

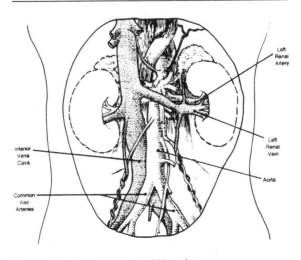

Figure 6-6 Normal Abdominal Vasculature

Palpation

The abdomen is palpated, tender quadrant last, for guarding, rigidity, organomegaly, tenderness, and the presence of a mass. Masses are characterized as to position, size, shape, consistency, and location. A fluid wave across the abdomen is consistent with ascites. Palpation for the abdominal aorta is a mandatory portion of this examination. Examination for hernia may also be performed at this juncture.

Percussion

The percussion note in each quadrant and over abdominal viscera is noted. The presence of shifting dullness with patient movement from right to left lateral decubitus positions is associated with ascites.

Hints

- Auscultation precedes palpation and percussion in the abdominal examination so as not to disturb bowel function before listening.
- A ticklish patient may be palpated with the patient's hand below the examiner's hand.
- Flexing the hips and knees while supine is the best position for examining the abdomen.
- Abdominal guarding is voluntary but rigidity is involuntary and suggests peritonitis.
- Lateral displacement of the fingers when palpating the aorta is consistent with aneurysm.
- The presence of a hard, nontender, immovable, left supraclavicular lymph node (Virchow's node) is often seen with metastatic gastrointestinal malignancy and lymphomas.
- Palpation of the popliteal fossa is mandatory in a patient suspected of having an abdominal aortic aneurysm, as many of these patients also have popliteal artery dilatation.

Extremities

Inspection

A check is made for any visible ulcers, varicosities, edema, atrophy, or deformity. Comparing right to left for symmetry is the best way to examine the extremities.

Palpation

Palpation of the joints for swelling, lumps and bumps, tenderness, and redness is performed. Any muscular tenderness is noted.

Percussion

This study is usually deferred.

Auscultation

Auscultation is reserved for any areas suspicious for vascular disease, tumor, or fracture.

Special Examinations

Examination of the breast and prostate are covered under procedures (Chapter 11). Orthopedic and neurologic examinations are covered in Chapters 7 and 8, respectively.

Special Tests/Signs in Physical Examination

The following list of tests and signs are commonly used in physical examination to help with differential diagnosis of some of the more common patient complaints.

- *Battle's Sign*—Demonstrates retro-auricular ecchymosis associated with basilar skull fracture.
- *Chvostek's Sign*—Tapping over the region of the facial nerve causes spasm of the facial muscles. This reaction is seen with hypocalcemic tetany.
- *Clubbing (digital)*—Bulbous enlargement of the tips of the fingers seen most often with lung cancer, although it may be seen with many chronic diseases.
- *Cullen's Sign*—Periumbilical ecchymosis consistent with intraperitoneal bleeding.
- *Homans' Sign*—Calf pain while squeezing the calf and forcibly dorsiflexing the foot. This sign is con-

sistent with thrombophlebitis and/or deep vein thrombosis.

- *Levine's Sign*—When a patient having a myocardial infarction or angina pectoris clenches the fist and holds it at the sternal region while complaining of pain in that region.

- *McBurney's Sign*—Tenderness at the site one-third the distance from the anterior superior iliac spine to the umbilicus, suggestive of appendicitis.

- *Murphy's Punch Test*—A sharp punch at the costovertebral angles that elicits pain in a patient with renal disease.

- *Murphy's Sign*—Sharp pain on deep inspiration and palpation of the inferior edge of the liver. Consistent with cholecystitis.

- *Obturator Sign*—When flexion and external rotation of the right hip causes pain in the right lower quadrant, suggestive of appendicitis.

- *Psoas Sign*—When extending and elevating the right leg with the patient prone produces pain in the right lower quadrant; found in patients with appendicitis.

- *Racoon Eyes*—Periorbital ecchymosis in a patient with a possible skull fracture.

- *Rust's Sign*—When patient supports head with both hands, as in cases of cervical spine trauma. This sign is consistent with a spinal fracture.

- *Splinter Hemorrhages*—Longitudinal hemorrhages in the nail beds consistent with subacute bacterial endocarditis.

BIBLIOGRAPHY

Bates, Barbara. 1979. *A guide to physical examination*. Philadelphia: J.B. Lippincott.

Berkow, Robert, ed. 1982. *The Merck manual of diagnosis and therapy*. 14th ed. Rahway, N.J.: Merck Sharp and Dohme Laboratories.

Krupp, M. ed. 1985. *Physicians handbook*. Los Altos, Calif.: Lange.

Prior, J., J. Silberstein, and J. Stang. 1981. *Physical diagnosis: The history and examination of the patient*. 6th ed. St. Louis: C.V. Mosby Co.

Schroeder, S., L. Tierney, and M. Krupp, eds. 1988. *Current medical diagnosis and treatment*. Norwalk, Conn.: Appleton & Lange.

Yearbook Medical Publishers. 1984. *400 self-assessment picture tests in clinical medicine*. Chicago: Yearbook Medical Publishers.

7

Orthopedics

INTRODUCTION

Orthopedics is the study of the skeletal system and related structures and the diseases that affect that system.

Orthopedic evaluation is an intergral part of the examination of every chiropractic patient. Although many of the tests used are nonspecific, in many cases a combination of positive findings can lead the physician to a diagnosis.

It should be remembered that the best clinical yield from an orthopedic test occurs when the test or maneuver reproduces or aggravates the patient's chief complaint. If performing the test causes pain different from the chief complaint, then the pain and its characteristics should be noted but the test, in most cases, should not be considered positive.

Another important aspect of orthopedic evaluation is the absence of an important positive finding, the so-called "pertinent negative." The absence of positive findings with certain tests suggests that certain disease processes do not exist. For this reason, if a test is found to be negative, it should be noted as such.

USEFUL ORTHOPEDIC TESTS

This section of tests is by no means exhaustive. It is instead a compilation of the tests most germane to chiropractic practice. It is not the purpose of this chapter to teach the proper performance of these tests. Many texts are available for that purpose. This chapter instead deals with the conditions that are associated with positive examination findings.

Adam's Position

If a scoliosis, which is noted in upright posture, disappears or decreases with forward flexion, it is said to indicate that the scoliosis is functional and not structural.

Adson's Test

If elevating the arm at the shoulder causes the radial pulse to be lost or diminished, it indicates thoracic outlet neurovascular compression syndrome.

Allen's Test

Thoracic outlet neurovascular compression syndrome should be ruled out in a patient whose palm fails or is slow to revascularize after pressure is released from the radial and/or ulnar arteries and after the arm, with a clenched fist, has been elevated. Radial and/or ulnar artery insufficiency also suggests a positive test.

Anterior Drawer Sign

The distal bone of the affected joint is distracted anteriorly and an estimation of stability compared to the other side is made. This test is used in many joints. When positive, it indicates ligamentous rupture with instability.

Apley's Tests (Knee)

Compression

Pain when compressing the lower leg into the knee joint with the patient prone and the knee flexed to 90 degrees indicates meniscal damage.

Distraction

Pain when distracting the lower leg from the knee with the patient prone and the knee flexed to 90 degrees is a positive test and indicates ligamentous damage.

Apparent Leg Length

The measurement from the umbilicus to the medial malleolus should be equal bilaterally. This test is non-specific for functional leg length inequality that is muscular or ligamentous in nature.

Bechterew's Test

A straight leg maneuver is performed with the patient seated. The test is positive when pain radiates down the posterior aspect of the leg. In most cases, this indicates some form of nerve root tension, usually from an intracanalicular space-occupying lesion.

Bowstring Sign

This is considered by some to be the sine qua non indicator of root tension from an intracanalicular space-occupying lesion, usually a herniated nucleus pulposus. The patient's leg is taken to the point of pain with a straight leg maneuver, after which the knee is slightly flexed and the foot allowed to rest on the examiner's shoulder until the pain subsides. Pressure is then placed in the popliteal fossa. Reproduction of pain down the leg is a positive sign while pain focally in the fossa is not.

Braggard's Test

The straight leg maneuver is performed and then the patient's foot is dorsiflexed. If positive, it confirms nerve root tension/irritation, although peripheral entrapment may also produce positive findings.

Brudzinski's Sign

The patient's head is forcibly flexed with the patient in the supine posture. Notation is made of flexion of both hips and both knees. Positive findings are consistent with meningeal irritation.

Codman's Sign

Rotator cuff tear/rupture should be suspected when the patient's arm is passively abducted above the horizontal and released, resulting in shoulder pain and elevation of the shoulder to compensate for loss of rotator cuff function.

Costoclavicular Tests

These maneuvers are indicative of thoracic outlet neurovascular compression syndrome. Any procedure that pulls the shoulders downwards and backwards and produces signs and symptoms of thoracic outlet syndrome should be regarded with suspicion.

Cozen's Test

If pain is felt while an attempt is made to flex the clenched fist, which is held in dorsiflexion, it indicates lateral epicondylitis or radiohumeral bursitis.

Dejerine's Triad

When coughing, sneezing, or straining at the stool, an intracanalicular space-occupying mass must be considered, when reproduction of pain and/or radiation of pain is present.

Distraction Test (Cervical Spine)

Axial distraction of the head away from the shoulders is performed. If pain is produced, myofascial disorders are the rule; if there is pain relief, foraminal encroachment should be suspected.

Dugas' Test

The patient places the hand of the affected side on the opposite shoulder. The inability to maintain this posture is significant for shoulder dislocation.

Ely's (Heel-To-Buttock) Test

The thigh is hyperextended after the knee has been flexed, with the patient in the prone position. Hip lesions, iliopsoas muscle irritation, and lumbar nerve root tension will cause positive findings.

Finklestein's Test

A positive test is consistent with stenosing tenosynovitis at the base of the thumb when the patient closes his or her fist around the thumb and then performs ulnar deviation at the wrist.

Gaenslen's Test

The patient, while in the supine position, is told to hold the unaffected side in the knee and hip-flexed position. The affected side is then lowered off the side of the table and pressure is placed on the knee of the extended leg. Positive findings are consistent with a sacroiliac lesion.

George's Vertebrobasilar Artery Tests

This group of tests is covered in Chapter 11.

Goldthwait's Test

This maneuver is used to differentiate lumbar spine from sacroiliac lesions. A straight leg raise maneuver is performed while the examiner places a hand under the lumbar spine. If pain is felt before the lumbar spine begins to move, a sacroiliac lesion is suspected. If the pain occurs after the lumbar spine begins to move, then a lumbar spine lesion is suspected.

Hibbs' Test

With the patient prone and the opposite side knee flexed to 90 degrees, the leg is rotated outward while the opposite side of the pelvis is stabilized. The location of any pain is noted. Depending on the site of pain, this test may be positive for sacroiliac and hip disease.

Homan's Sign

This test indicates thrombophlebitis or deep vein thrombosis when pain is felt deep in the calf of the leg where the foot is forcibly dorsiflexed with the knee fully extended.

Iliac Compression

With the patient in side posture, downward pressure is placed on the pelvis and the location of pain is noted. Depending upon the site of pain, positive findings in this test indicate either pelvic or sacroiliac disease/lesion.

Jackson's Compression Test

With the neck laterally flexed, rotated, and extended, downward pressure is placed on the top of the head. Positive findings indicate nerve root compression or facet pathology in the cervical spine.

Kemp's Test

This is a relatively nonspecific test for lumbar spine disorders, with an emphasis on posterior vertebral column disease or disc herniation. With the patient standing, the lumbar spine is laterally flexed, rotated, and extended. An attempt is then made by the examiner to exaggerate this posture. The nature and location of pain is noted.

Kernig's Sign

While the patient is supine, the knee and hip on one side are flexed to 90 degrees and then the knee is fully extended. A positive test indicates either meningitis or a radiculoneuropathy.

Lasègue's Test (Straight Leg Raising)

With the patient supine, the leg on the affected side is raised with the knee fully extended. This is a relatively nonspecific test for lumbar spine disease or peripheral neuropathy, although it may also produce pain with simple muscle spasm in the posterior thigh or leg.

Lewin's Test

With the patient standing, one knee at a time and then both knees together are rapidly pulled into hyperextension. This test can be positive with nerve root tension, peripheral neuropathy, or hamstring spasm/contracture.

Lindner's Sign

With the patient supine, the head, neck, and trunk are forced into flexion by the examiner elevating the body while grasping the occiput. Presence of this sign is consistent with nerve root tension or meningeal irritation (diffuse pain).

Maximum Cervical Compression Test

The neck is laterally flexed and then the chin is rotated to the same side of lateral flexion. The examiner may then place downward pressure on top of the head. A positive test can indicate either neural foraminal encroachment or posterior spinal column pathology.

McMurray's Test

The knee is extended to anatomical position after the foot of the affected side has been approximated to the buttock and the hip externally rotated. Depending on the position of the knee during testing, a click that is heard or felt can indicate either medial or lateral meniscus pathology.

Milgram's Test

This is a relatively nonspecific test for low back pathology. While the patient is supine, both feet are lifted off the table and an attempt is made to hold the feet approximately 6 inches off the table.

Mill's Test

Pain felt when the arm is pronated with a fully extended elbow and flexed wrist and fingers indicates lateral epicondylitis.

Minor's Sign

This motion (using the arms to raise from a chair while flexing at the hips to protect the low back) is classically found in patients with true nerve root tension.

Neri's Bowing Test

The patient attempts to flex forward from the standing position without bending the knees. If the knees are bent during the maneuver, it is a sign of nerve root tension, peripheral neuropathy, or hamstring spasm.

Ober's Test

The patient lies in side posture and the leg is abducted at the hip. After the examiner releases his or her grasp on the leg, it should fall back to neutral position. If it remains passively abducted, test findings are considered positive. A positive test classically indicates an iliotibial band (abduction) contracture at the hip.

Ortolani's Click Test

If a click is heard or felt when abducting an infant's hips with the hips and knees flexed, it is a sign of congenital dislocation of the hip.

Patrick Fabere Test (Figure Four Test)

This test has been classically associated with hip joint disease. The affected hip is flexed, abducted, and externally rotated and further abduction pressure is placed at the knee.

Shoulder Depression Test

The head is laterally flexed and the shoulder depressed with the patient in the supine posture. This test may produce pain with a number of lesions, including brachial plexus disorders, nerve root tension, muscle spasm, and posterior spinal column disease.

Soto-Hall Test

With the patient supine, the examiner flexes the neck with one hand while placing the other hand on the sternum to prevent flexion of any of the rest of the spine. Positive findings in this test have classically been associated with compression fractures, but may be seen with most any vertebral disease, including nerve root tension.

Spinous Percussion

This test is used to facilitate localization of spinal pathology.

Spurling's Maneuver

The patient's head is maximally rotated and extended and downward pressure is placed on the top of the head and/or a blow to the top of the head is given. This test may yield positive findings in instances of nerve root tension and/or posterior joint disease.

Thomas Test

The examiner fully flexes the knee and hip on the unaffected side and notes whether the opposite leg moves into a similar but less pronounced posture. Positive findings in this test typically indicate hip flexion contracture, although they may also occur with flexor spasm.

Thompson's Test

With the patient prone, the examiner squeezes the calf muscles. Normally there is plantarflexion of the foot with this maneuver. This test is diagnostic of an Achilles's tendon rupture.

Trendelenburg's Test

The patient stands and lifts one foot off the floor. Normally the pelvis on the same side will elevate as well. If it fails to elevate, the test is considered positive. Positive findings in this test are classically associated with gluteus medius/hip abductor weakness.

Tripod Sign

This sign can be seen with anything from hamstring spasm to true nerve root tension, from the thoracic spine caudally. If the seated patient leans back and supports the upper body with the arms while the legs are being extended, the test is considered positive.

Valgus and Varus Stress

These two maneuvers are used to indicate ligamentous stability in a number of different joints.

Valsalva Maneuver

The patient bears down as if he or she is having a bowel movement. A positive test indicates intracanalicular space-occupying lesions.

Wright's Hyperabduction Test

When the extended arm is hyperabducted, the radial pulse should remain intact at the same degree bilaterally. Premature loss of the pulse is consistent with thoracic outlet neurovascular compression syndromes.

Yeoman's Test

While the patient is prone, the examiner fully flexes the knee to the buttock and then hyperextends the hip while placing pressure on the sacroiliac joint. Pain production is consistent with sacroiliac joint disease, especially sprain of the anterior sacroiliac ligaments.

Yergason's Test

With the seated patient's elbow at 90 degrees of flexion, resisted pronation and supination of the wrist are performed. Pain and/or clicking in the bicipital groove with resisted supination is a positive test. Positive findings are classically associated with biceps tendon lesions, including instability.

RANGE OF MOTION

The assessment of joint range of motion is an especially important portion of the orthopedic examination for chiropractic clinicians. Restoration of joint range of motion is a major goal of therapy in most cases. Table 7-1 contains a list of the ranges of motion

Table 7-1 Assessing Range of Motion

Body Part	Motion	Range of Motion
Ankle	Dorsiflexion	15–20
	Plantarflexion	40–50
	Inversion	05
	Eversion	05
Cervical Spine	Extension	40–50
	Flexion	40–50
	Lateral bending	40–50
	Rotation	40–60
Elbow	Flexion	140–150
	Extension	00
Fingers	Flexion	
	Distal interphalangeal joint	70–90
	Proximal interphalangeal joint	90–100
	Metacarpophalangeal joint	85–95
	Extension	00–05
Forearm	Pronation	60–80
	Supination	80–90
Forefoot	Eversion	15–20
	Inversion	30–35
Hip	Abduction	45–50
	Adduction	20–30
	Extension	25–35
	Flexion	110–120
	Rotation (external)	40–50
	Rotation (internal)	30–40
Knee	Extension	00–10
	Flexion	85–95
	Lateral bending	15–25
	Rotation	25–35
Shoulder	Abduction	170–180
	Adduction	40–50
	Extension	40–50
	Flexion	170–180
	Rotation (external)	80–90
	Rotation (internal)	70–90
Toes	First metatarsophalangeal joint	
	Extension	70–90
	Flexion	40–45
Wrist	Extension	60–70
	Flexion	70–80
	Radial deviation	15–20
	Ulnar deviation	25–30

for the various joints of the body. Range of motion is most accurately measured with a goniometer.

SCOLIOSIS EVALUATION

Only a thorough evaluation of patients with scoliosis can accurately assess which of the many types of available therapy will best fit the needs of the patient. The etiology of scoliosis is just as important as the degree of deformity in determining appropriate treatment. Proper evaluation includes an appropriate history, physical examination, and radiography of the spine.

History

Other family members should be assessed for a history of scoliosis. The cause of the scoliosis should be sought, especially if it is a dysplastic cause, such as neurofibromatosis or Marfan's syndrome. The patient should then be examined for any findings of these syndromes.

Physical Examination

The evaluating physician should measure the lateral and posterior curvatures of the spine, as well as the rib hump, shoulder, and pelvic heights. These measurements will serve as reference points for future examinations and for charting the progression or regression of the curvatures.

Examination of the thorax is of paramount importance in scoliosis patients. Many patients with severe curvatures suffer from cardiovascular and pulmonary disease secondary to reduced thoracic cage volume.

An entire head-to-toe physical examination should also be completed, with special emphasis on the rate of growth if the patient is not a skeletally mature adult. Follow-up examinations are imperative in charting the patient's progress. These may be performed as often as weekly if, in the clinical judgment of the physician, it will be of benefit to the patient.

A number of nonradiographic tools are available for the evaluation of scoliosis, including plumb line analysis, bilateral scales, and a scoliometer to measure rib hump size.

Radiographic Examination

Full spine anteroposterior and sometimes lateral radiographic examination of the spine is essential in any patient suspected of having scoliosis. The lateral and anteroposterior curvatures of the spine are measured and recorded for future reference (Figures 7-1 and 7-2). An estimation of the patient's skeletal age is also made (Figure 7-3). This measurement will assist

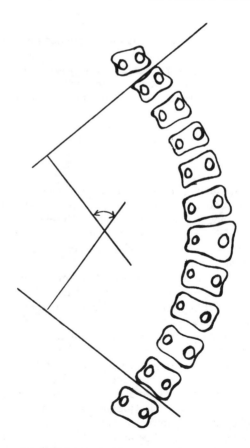

Figure 7-1 Cobb Method of Scoliosis Measurement

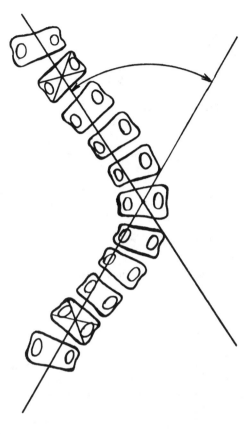

Figure 7-2 Risser-Ferguson Method of Scoliosis Measurement

---

in the prediction of any future progression of the curvature(s).

Treatment

The treatment of scoliosis varies from simple exercises to surgical intervention. The type of treatment varies with the type and severity of the curvature, the age of the patient, and any associated visceral abnormalities. Most curvatures seen in chiropractic general practice can be managed with manipulation, exercise, stretching, muscle stimulation, and bracing. Proper brace requisition and fitting are best accomplished by

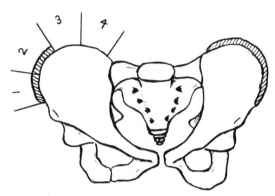

Note: After grade 4 and the apophysis fuses, skeletal growth has ceased.

Figure 7-3 Risser's Sign of Skeletal Maturation

referral to an orthotist with instructions from the treating physician.

SPONDYLOLISTHESIS

Spondylolisthesis (SL) is the abnormal anterior translation of a vertebral body associated with lesions or deformity of the posterior arch of the involved vertebra. It has been somewhat of an enigma for all the health care disciplines for many years. Treatment regimens vary from rest to forms of radical surgery. As yet, no one has arrived at any definitive conclusions as to the etiology, let alone, treatment of SL.

This section will discuss theories regarding pathogenesis, proper diagnosis, and chiropractic treatment as well as surgical management of SL.

Pathogenesis

There are five basic etiologies for SL (listed in Exhibit 7-1). The most common form of SL is *spondylolytic*. In this form, there is a stress fracture at the pars interarticularis of the vertebral arch, which results in anterolisthesis of the involved vertebra. This type of SL occurs most commonly at L5 but may also be seen anywhere throughout the spine. Pain is usually present at the level above the lesion and there may or may not be radiation into the buttock(s) and leg(s).

Exhibit 7-1 Types of Spondylolisthesis

Spondylolytic
Degenerative
Congenital
Traumatic
Dysplastic

Degenerative SL, on the other hand, does not involve fracture of any portion of the vertebral body. Its presentation is that of an anterolisthesis of a vertebral body at the level of a degenerated disc and many times unusual facet joint morphology and facet arthrosis. There is a conspicuous absence of pars defects with this form of SL.

Traumatic SL is usually reserved for fractured pedicles at C2 from severe hyperextension injuries of the neck. This form of SL may present to the chiropractic office. Care should be taken to rule out its presence in a trauma patient before any manipulation is performed, lest neurologic sequelae possibly result.

Congenital and *dysplastic SL* are uncommon and the reader is referred to more in-depth texts on the subject.

Diagnosis

The diagnosis of SL is usually straightforward when radiography is employed; the main question is the etiology of the SL. The presence or absence of pars defects characterizes spondylolytic and degenerative types, respectively. Oblique radiographic views confirm this distinction. Traumatic SL occurs most commonly in the cervical spine and is associated with severe hyperextension injuries.

If there is a possibility of instability, then flexion and extension radiographic views and hanging or compression radiography may be helpful. Additional anterolisthesis during these special maneuvers may be suggestive of instability and may require referral if the patient is significantly affected or incapacitated by the pain or has neurological defects.

Treatment

Although treatment is multifaceted, it appears that manipulation and exercise that somehow reduces the anterior curve of the lumbar spine functions well for pain reduction (barring any contraindications to manipulation). Surgical intervention usually involves arthrodesis with or without a laminectomy. The reader is referred to more in-depth texts for further treatment protocols.

SCREENING EXAMINATIONS

After the patient's chief complaint is recorded and established as either an orthopedic or a neurological problem, a screening examination may be performed to help the clinician isolate the area of the problem so that a more detailed examination of that area may be performed. It should be remembered that these screening examinations in no way specifically isolate the diagnosis. It should also be remembered that visceral pathology can refer pain to any area of the musculoskeletal system. There are two screening exams; the upper body and lower body screening examinations.

Upper Body Screening Examination (with patient sitting)

- Inspection
  —Head and neck
  —Shoulders
  —Elbows
  —Wrists
  —Hands
- Shoulder range of motion
  —Active abduction with end of range pressure (EORP)
  —Active extension with adduction with EORP
- Cervical spine
  —Active ranges of motion
  —Passive motion with EORP
  —Resisted range of motion (Exhibit 7-2)
  —Vertebrobasilar artery patency tests

Exhibit 7-2 Upper Body Muscle Testing

> Cervical flexion/extension
> Elbow flexion
> Shoulder rotation/abduction
> Wrist flexion/extension
> Finger squeeze

- Dermatomes/sensory
  —Pinwheel examination (with two instruments)
  —Sensation of pins/needles/numbness/tingling
- Reflexes
  —Biceps brachialis (C5)
  —Brachioradialis (C6)
  —Triceps (C7)
  —Detailed evaluation of area of involvement suggested by the screening examination

Lower Body Screening Examination

- Patient standing
  —Posture
  —Deep knee bend (tests all joints of lower extremity)
  —Tandem gait (away from examiner) (ataxia?)
  —Heel walk (towards examiner) (L4/5)
  —Toe walk (away from examiner) (L5/S_1)
- Patient sitting
  —Thoracolumbar spine
      Inspection
      Active range of motion with EORP
      Passive range of motion with EORP
  —Orthopedic tests
      Valsalva Maneuver
      Internal rotation of the hip
  —Neurological tests
      Dermatomes (bilateral with pinwheels)
      Reflexes
        Knee jerk (L3/4)
        Ankle jerk (S1)
- Patient supine
  —Orthopedic tests
      Sciatic nerve stretch tests

Exhibit 7-3 Lower Body Muscle Testing

Lumbar flexion/extension
Hip flexion/extension
Knee flexion/extension
Ankle dorsiflexion/plantar flexion
Great toe extension

Patrick Fabere test
—Hip evaluation
    Active range of motion with EORP
    Passive range of motion with EORP
—Knee evaluation
    Active range of motion with EORP
    Passive range of motion with EORP
    Valgus/varus stress
—Ankle evaluation
    Active range of motion with EORP
    Passive range of motion with EORP
    Anterior/posterior drawer sign
—Reflexes
    Babinski response (upper motor neuron lesion)
    Shin tracing with heel (cerebellar integrity)
• Patient prone
—Gluteal mass inspection
—Orthopedic tests
    Femoral nerve stretch tests
    Internal/external hip rotation
    Spring test (SI joint)
—Resisted muscle testing (Exhibit 7-3)
• Detailed evaluation of the area of involvement suggested by the screening examination

---

BIBLIOGRAPHY

Rammamurti, C. 1979. *Orthopedics in primary care*. Baltimore: Williams & Wilkins Co.

Turek, J. 1988. *Orthopedics: Principles and their application*. Philadelphia: J.B. Lippincott.

8

Neurologic Evaluation

INTRODUCTION

Neurology is the study of diseases that affect the nervous system. For many years, the beneficial and detrimental effects of manipulation on the human nervous system have been investigated by researchers. Recent findings better explain those effects. It is known that complications, particularly involving postmanipulative inflammation, vascular damage, and hemorrhage and ischemic neurological sequelae, may occur with chiropractic manipulation in extremely rare instances. These sequelae range from continued pain to quadriplegia and, in some extremely rare cases, death.

This chapter concerns the neurologic evaluation of patients presenting to the chiropractic physician. Emphasis is placed on diagnostics and the evaluation of the patient for neurologic contraindications to manipulation.

The neurologic evaluation of a patient is divided into four separate parts: location of the lesion, etiology of the lesion, treatment of the lesion, and contraindications to manipulation because of the lesion.

LOCATION OF THE LESION

An important aspect of neurodiagnosis that concerns the chiropractor is locating the lesion. In most instances, the location of the lesion defines treatment and helps define any contraindications to manipulation.

The first step in locating the lesion is to decide whether it involves the central nervous system (CNS) or peripheral nervous system (PNS), i.e., whether the lesion is an upper motor neuron lesion (UMNL) or lower motor neuron lesion (LMNL) (see Table 8-1). This decision is based on a number of different findings resulting from evaluation of the deep tendon reflexes (DTR), type of paralysis/paresis, presence of fasciculations/fibrillations, presence of atrophy, and the Babinski reflex.

Deep Tendon Reflexes

Hyperreflexia is consistent with an UMNL and hyporeflexia with an LMNL. Reflexes are graded from 0 to +4 (see Table 8-2). Clonus, or rapid involuntary alternating movements, may also be present with an UMNL.

Paralysis/Paresis

Spastic paralysis is suggestive of an UMNL while flaccid paralysis is consistent with an LMNL. Spastic paralysis is hallmarked by an inability to move an extremity, both voluntarily and involuntarily. Muscle rigidity prevents, or at least restricts, passive motion and may even result in the so-called "cogwheel" response. This lesion appears as a jerky motion when the extremity is passively moved.

Fasciculations or Fibrillations

Fasciculations are palpable involuntary muscle contractions and fibrillations are invisible muscle contractions. These contractions are seen with an LMNL.

Table 8-1 Upper versus Lower Motor Neuron Lesions

Test	UMNL	LMNL
Paralysis	Spastic	Flaccid
Atrophy	+/−	+
Babinski	+	−
Clonus	+	−
DTRs	+	−
Fasciculation	−	+

Note: + = increased; − = decreased.

Table 8-2 Deep Tendon Reflex Grading

Grade	Explanation
0	No reflex
+1	Mildly decreased
+2	Normal
+3	Mildly increased
+4	Hyperactive

Atrophy or Babinski Reflex

Atrophy is consistent with an LMNL while a Babinski response (dorsiflexion of the great toe with spreading of the lateral four toes upon stroking the plantar surface of the foot) is diagnostic of an UMNL. It should be remembered that children under the age of one will have a positive Babinski response under normal circumstances since their CNS is still developing.

If the lesion is determined to be an LMNL, it must then be decided if the defect is at the nerve root or in the peripheral nerve. Nerve root lesions are suggested by positive orthopedic tests for nerve root tension. Pain in a root lesion will also be noted from the spine to below the elbow or knee in a dermatomal pattern, whereas the pain and numbness of a peripheral lesion begins at the site of entrapment and does not follow a dermatomal pattern. Pain is less often seen with peripheral lesions. Dermatomes are illustrated in Figure 8-1.

If the lesion is determined to involve the CNS it must then be decided whether the spinal cord or brain is the primary site of the lesion (see Table 8-3).

Spinal Cord Lesions

Spinal cord lesions will typically present with UMNL findings, along with a dermatomal defect and dissociation of sensory function in the extremities. Dissociation is the separation of sensory losses to opposite sides of the body. For example, if pain and temperature sensation are lost on one side of the body and proprioception on the contralateral side, the patient must have a spinal cord lesion. Only with this location do the sensory tracts cross to the contralateral side.

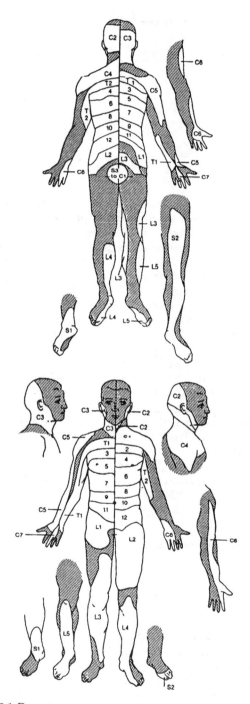

Figure 8-1 Dermatomes

Table 8-3 Brain versus Spinal Cord Lesion

Brain	Spinal Cord
UMNL	UMNL
CN deficits	Dermatomal deficit
Contralateral sensory loss	Dissociation of sensory function

Brain Lesions

In lesions of the brain, sensory losses would be on the contralateral side.

If there is cranial nerve deficit, then the lesion must be above the foramen magnum. The same holds true if there is ipsilateral loss of pain and temperature and proprioception along with a hemiplegia.

After the lesion is isolated to above the foramen magnum, it must further be located either above or below the tentorium cerebelli (see Table 8-4). Infratentorial lesions involve the cerebellum or brain stem and supratentorial lesions involve the cerebrum.

If a cranial nerve deficit is contralateral to the side of hemiparesis or hemiplegia, then the brain stem must be involved. Lesions of the cerebrum will cause both of these deficits on the same side of the body and in many cases will not cause cranial nerve palsies because of crossover of their nerve fibers.

Cortical lesions are also hallmarked by altered mental status, such as loss of recent memory, personality changes, aphasia, the inability to speak, and complete inability to perform normal motor tasks.

Cerebellar lesions tend to produce ipsilateral loss while cerebral lesions produce contralateral deficit. Basal ganglia lesions also tend to produce resting tremors while cerebellar lesions produce intention tremors.

ETIOLOGY OF THE LESION

Now that the lesion has been located, the cause of the problem needs to be isolated. The list of etiologies

Table 8-4 Supratentorial versus Infratentorial Lesions

Supratentorial	Infratentorial
Contralateral hemiplegia and CN deficit(s)	Ipsilateral hemiplegia and CN deficit(s)
Altered mental status	Normal mentation

responsible for neurologic disease is far too extensive
to be covered in this text. (The reader is referred to the
bibliography at the end of this chapter for in-depth
discussion.) Instead, this chapter will cover the causes
of neurologic lesions most commonly seen in chiropractic practice.

Peripheral Lesions

The most common peripheral nerve lesions are
listed in Exhibit 8-1. Diabetes mellitus often can cause
peripheral polyneuropathy, especially that affecting
the hands and feet, the so-called "glove and stocking"
paresthesias. Historical confirmation is made by af-
firming the presence of excessive thirst, hunger, and
urination. Serum hyperglycemia is the indicator of
diabetes mellitus.

Peripheral nerve compression syndromes are common in clinical practice. Diseases such as carpal tunnel
syndrome and thoracic outlet syndrome are diag-
nosed by orthopedic and neurological testing. The
presence of muscle atrophy is most often an ominous
sign; in such instances, a neurosurgical consultation
may be helpful.

Nerve Root Lesions

Common nerve root lesions are listed in Exhibit 8-2.
The most often seen is compression by a herniated disc
with signs and symptoms of a radiculopathy (Exhibit 8-3). Encroachment of an intervertebral foramen
by either fibrosis or osteophytes causes a similar picture. Herpes zoster (shingles) and tabes dorsalis
(neurosyphilis) can also result in nerve root
involvement.

Exhibit 8-1 Common Peripheral Nerve Lesions

Diabetic neuropathy
Thoracic outlet syndrome
Carpal tunnel syndrome
Tarsal tunnel syndrome
Brachial plexus syndromes

Exhibit 8-2 Common Nerve Root Lesions

Herniated nucleus pulposus
Disc bulge
Dural sleeve adhesions
Osseous foraminal encroachment
Lateral recess stenosis

Spinal Cord Lesions

There are a number of spinal cord lesions (listed in Exhibit 8-4) that can present with the signs and symptoms noted above. These include the Brown-Séquard syndrome (hemisection of the cord); central disc herniations and tumors, which can result in the cauda equina syndrome; transection of the cord; and diseases intrinsic to the spinal cord, such as metastasis and syringomyelia.

Brain Stem Lesions

Lesions of the brain stem (medulla, pons, and midbrain) are usually from either vascular disease or tumor. Common tumors of the brain stem include gliomas, acoustic neuromas, and meningiomas (see also Exhibit 8-5).

Cerebral Lesions

Vascular diseases (such as ischemia, hemorrhage, and aneurysms) along with tumors (especially gliomas) are the most common cerebral lesions (see also Exhibit 8-6).

Exhibit 8-3 Signs and Symptoms of Radiculopathy

Dermatomal pain (past elbow/knee)
Atrophy
Decreased deep tendon reflexes
Fasciculations/fibrillations

Exhibit 8-4 Common Spinal Cord Lesions

Central HNP
Metastasis
Syringomyelia
Brown-Séquard Syndrome
Spinal Canal Stenosis

Exhibit 8-5 Common Brain Stem Lesions

Vascular
  Ischemia
  Arteriovenous malformation
  Aneurysm
Neoplasm
  Gliomas
  Acoustic neuroma
  Meningioma

TREATMENT OF THE LESION AND CONTRAINDICATIONS TO TREATMENT

Most often, the treatment of a true neurologic lesion with acute paralysis, atrophy, and other ominous signs will be undertaken by a neurologist or neurosurgeon.

One of the main thrusts of diagnosis by the chiropractic clinician is to rule out the possibility of CNS lesions, surgical cases, and contraindications to manip-

Exhibit 8-6 Common Cerebral Lesions

Vascular
  Hemorrhage
  Ischemia
  Aneurysm
Neoplasm
  Gliomas
    Astrocytoma
    Glioblastoma multiforme

ulation. For example, the chiropractic doctor will most often treat patients' nonsurgical neurologic lesions, such as disc herniations. However, if a herniation causes a cauda equina syndrome or the patient has atrophy, fasciculations, muscle weakness, or paralysis, the patient should be referred for neurosurgical consultation.

Challenges to the carotid and vertebrobasilar artery systems for patency must be performed on all patients undergoing cervical spine manipulation. When those systems are compromised, aggressive dynamic manipulation of the patient's neck is contraindicated and referral to a vascular or neurological surgeon for more extensive investigation is required.

There are many neurologic diseases that chiropractors treat frequently and with much success, such as herniated nucleus pulposi and peripheral nerve entrapments. It is beyond the scope of this text to outline treatment protocols for the many neurologic lesions. The reader is referred to other chapters in this book for the investigation and treatment of cervical spine and low back pain.

Neurological/Neurosurgical Consultation

Consultation with a neurologist or neurosurgeon should be sought for a number of neurologic lesions. The reason for referral is not always for treatment but for advanced evaluation and legal protection of the chiropractic doctor. Consultation should be sought for the following conditions:

- Cauda Equina Syndrome
- Cerebrovascular Accident
- CNS Tumors
- Vertebrobasilar Artery Insufficiency
- Cerebral Aneurysm
- Subarachnoid Hemorrhage
- Muscle Atrophy
- Fasciculations/Fibrillations
- Positive Babinski Sign

Screening Neurologic Examination

The following list is a quick screening examination of the nervous system. It should not replace an in-depth evaluation of patients who present with a primary neurologic complaint.

- *Mental Status Examination*—Counting in serial reverse sevens, counting backwards from 100 by sevens; describing orientation with regard to person, place, time, and situation; and recalling objects at the end of the exam are appropriate screening tools for assessing mental status.
- *Cranial Nerve Examination*—The cranial nerves are tested as follows:
  II—Near/far visual acuity
  III, IV, VI—Cardinal ranges of motion of the eyes, pupillary response
  V—Light touch on the face, corneal reflex
  VII—Smile/frown
  VIII—Listen for finger rubbing
  IX, X—Gag reflex
  XI—Elevate the shoulders
  XII—Protrude the tongue
- *Reflexes*—When the Babinski reflex (stroking the bottom of the foot) elicits fanning of the lateral four toes and dorsiflexion of the great toe, this is the sign of an upper motor neuron lesion. Deep tendon reflexes should also be performed.
- *Sensory Examination*—Bilateral pinprick and vibrations sense should be compared for symmetry and dissociation of senses.
- *Motor Examination*—Resisted flexion and extension ranges of motion and finger squeeze and great toe extension are tested and graded (Table 8-5).

Table 8-5 Muscle Strength Grading System

Grade	Explanation
0	No muscle contraction
+1	Visible fasciculations
+2	Slight muscle contraction
+3	Movement with no gravity
+4	Movement against slight resistance
+5	Movement against full gravity

- *Cerebellar Challenge*—Romberg test, finger to nose, and finger to doctor's moving finger are screening tests for cerebellar function.

BIBLIOGRAPHY

Dejong, R. 1979. *The neurologic examination.* New York: Harper & Row.

Dornbrand, L., A. Hoole, R. Fletcher, and G. Pickard. 1985. *Manual of clinical problems in adult ambulatory care.* Boston: Little, Brown & Co.

Thurston, S., ed. 1987. *The little black book of neurology.* Chicago: Yearbook Medical Publishers.

9

Laboratory Diagnosis

INTRODUCTION

Laboratory diagnosis is essential in evaluating patient complaints. It has, unfortunately, in recent years become more of a "crutch" than an adjunct to good history taking and physical examination procedures.

Clinical laboratory tests can be vital tools for arriving at a final diagnosis, excluding pathology, and performing screening tests. This chapter outlines clinical laboratory diagnosis by defining tests that are useful in chiropractic practice. If a decreased or increased value is not clinically useful (i.e., it has a low sensitivity and specificity), it has been excluded from this text.

Many facilities offer a panel of tests (e.g., SMA 12, CHEM 23) that are performed on a single sample. Physicians should investigate their facilities to learn the standard protocols.

The values listed in this chapter are for general use. Specific ranges are usually included on the reports from each institution. Unless otherwise specified, the listed values are for the adult patient. (A list of helpful shorthand terms for laboratory values can be found in Figure 9-1.)

COMPLETE BLOOD COUNT (CBC)

The complete blood count includes the red blood cell (RBC) count, white blood cell (WBC) count, hemo-

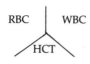

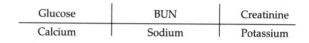

| Glucose | BUN | Creatinine |
| Calcium | Sodium | Potassium |

Figure 9-1 Laboratory Shorthand

globin (Hgb), hematocrit (Hct), mean cellular volume (MCV), mean corpuscular hemoglobin (MCH), mean corpuscular hemoglobin concentration (MCHC), and a platelet count. The breakdown of different types of WBCs (differential) may be included or may have to be ordered separately. (Normal CBC values are listed in Table 9-1.)

Blood Smear with Wright's Stain

This procedure is used for manually determining the WBC differential count.

Performing the Smear

1. Place a single drop of blood from the anticoagulated tube (purple top) in the center of a clean

Table 9-1 CBC Normal Values

Blood Component	Value
Red blood cells	3.9–5.2 million/mm³
White blood cells	3,800–10,000/mm³
Neutrophils	40–75%
Lymphocytes	18–47%
Eosinophils	0–6%
Basophils	0–2%
Monocytes	0–10%
Hemoglobin	12–16 gm/dL (female)
	14–18 gm/dL (male)
Hematocrit	35–47% (female)
	40–55% (male)
Platelets	130,000–400,000/mm³

slide approximately 1 inch from the end of the slide.

2. Use the "spreading slide" to smear the original sample by placing the "smearing slide" at a 45 degree angle to the original and bringing it to the edge of the blood drop. The drop will then spread along the edge of the tilted slide. As soon as this dispersion occurs, quickly move the tilted slide away from the drop. This will form a thin film of blood across the original slide, which is approximately 3 centimeters long.

3. Check to insure that the film of blood is thin and of uniform thickness. RBCs should be evenly distributed along the length of the smear.

Staining the Slide

1. Let the slide dry (preferably air dry). Mark the patient's name and the date on the slide in pencil.

2. Fix the slide for one minute in methanol. Do not rinse or dry the slide after it has been fixed.

3. Place the slide in the Wright's stain for 30 to 90 seconds.

4. Remove the slide, rinse it with tap water, and let it air dry. The slide is ready for viewing.

Viewing the Slide

1. The portion of the slide where the RBCs are in close approximation but do not overlap is the best place to examine for cells.

2. Examine a strip along the central portion of the slide. Avoid the edges and ends of the smear as the cell count will be skewed with this technique. Examination should be performed with oil immersion.

3. The white cell counter available in most laboratories is an excellent tool for counting the differential.

The remaining counts in the CBC are usually made with an automated cell counter although the RBC indices (MCV, MCH, and MCHC) can be done from the RBC, Hct, and Hgb with a special calculator.

Interpreting the CBC (common normal values are in parentheses)

Red Blood Cell Count (male = 3.9–5.2 million/mm³)

Decrease: Anemias

Increase: Polycythemias, high altitudes

Note: The most common form of anemia is caused by iron deficiency. Any anemia in a patient over 40 is from a gastrointestinal malignancy until proven otherwise. Follow up with rectal exam, testing for occult blood in the stool and serum iron.

Red Blood Cell Morphology

Anisocytosis: Irregular size of red blood cells. Anemias can present as normocytic, microcytic (iron deficiency), and macrocytic (megaloblastic anemia). This parameter is measured as mean cellular volume (MCV).

Poikilocytosis: Irregular shape of red blood cells. Examples include:

Sickling—sickle cell anemia

Nucleated—marrow replacement, hemorrhage extramedullary hematopoiesis

Acanthocytes (burr cells)—liver disease

Target cells—any hypochromic anemia

Cellular inclusions: Basophilic stippling—heavy metal poisoning

Howell-Jolly bodies—postsplenectomy

Mean Corpuscular Hemoglobin (27–33 picograms)

Decrease: Hypochromic anemias (iron deficiency)

Increase: Hyperchromic anemias (megaloblastic)

White Blood Cell Count (3,800–10,000/mm³)

Decrease: Chronic infections

Increase: Infections

White Blood Cell Differential

Segmented neutrophils = 40%–75%

Lymphocytes = 18%–47%

Eosinophils = 0%–6%

Basophils = 0%–2%

Monocytes = 0%–10%

Hemoglobin (male = 14–18 gm/dL; female 12–16 gm/dL)

Decrease: Anemias

Increase: Not usually seen
Hematocrit (male = 40%–55%; female = 35%–47%)
Decrease: Anemias, hemorrhage
Increase: Hemoconcentration, polycythemias
Platelets (130,000–400,000/mm³)
Decrease: Thrombocytopenia syndromes, leukemias
Increase: Not usually seen

URINALYSIS

The urinalysis (UA) is composed of the following tests. Normal adult values are noted parenthetically. Abnormal findings and their clinical significance are noted below each test. (Table 9-2 summarizes the tests and their normal values.)

Appearance (straw/clear)
Blue (or green)—beets
Brown—bile, hemoglobin, blood, food dyes
Cloudy (turbid)—phosphated, urates, WBCs
Dark (black)—porphyrins, melanin pigmentation
Foamy—protein, bile acids
Red—blood

Specific Gravity (1.01–1.03)
The specific gravity of the urine is an indirect reflection of the kidney's ability to concentrate urine. If the first morning specimen has specific gravity of 1.025 or better, it is a good indication of adequate concentration by the kidneys.

Decrease: Intrinsic renal disease, diabetes insipidus
Increase: Diabetes mellitus, congestive heart failure (CHF), nephrosis (proteinuria)
Ph (4.5–8.0)

Table 9-2 Normal Urinalysis

Characteristic	Value
Appearance	straw/clear
Specific gravity	1.01–1.03
Ph	4.5–8.0
Glucose	negative
Ketones	negative
Blood	negative
Nitrites	negative
Bilirubin	negative
Urobilinogen	negative

Acid urine: Ketoacidosis, chronic obstructive pulmonary disease (COPD), high protein diet, medications

Alkaline urine: UTI, renal tubular acidosis, vomiting, high vegetable diet

Glucose (negative)

Normal urine never contains glucose, as the renal threshold before the glucose "spills over" into the urine is 180 mg%. If glucose is found in the urine, a diagnosis of diabetes mellitus should be entertained.

Positive: Diabetes mellitus, Cushing's syndrome, steroids, hyperthyroidism, pancreatic disease, renal tubular disease

Ketones (negative)

Positive: Diabetic ketoacidosis, vomiting, diarrhea, pregnancy, hyperthyroidism, starvation, high fat diet

Blood (negative)

If the dipstick is positive for blood but no cells are seen, there may be hemoglobin in the urine. Causes such as trauma should be sought.

Positive: Infection, stones, trauma, tumors. False positive in athletes from repetitive microtrauma.

Nitrites (negative)

Positive: Urinary tract infection (UTI) (except when organism does not produce nitrites; therefore, a negative test does not rule out infection)

Bilirubin (negative)

Positive: Multiple myeloma, UTI, genitourinary (GU) malignancy, CHF, preeclampsia, malignant hypertension (HTN)

Urobilinogen (0.1–1.0 mg/dL)

Increase: Cirrhosis, right-sided CHF, hepatitis, antibiotic therapy

All of the above tests, except the appearance of the urine, can be performed by the dipstick method with a freshly voided specimen. After the dipstick analysis is performed, the urine must be examined microscopically for the presence of cells, casts, and bacteria. Table 9-3 lists the casts found in urine and the clinical significance of each.

Culture and sensitivity to antibiotics may be in order for a patient with a suspected urinary tract infection. Gram staining of bacteria may also be performed. A urinalysis with gram staining and culture should be

Table 9-3 Urine Casts

Cast	Significance
Waxy	Advanced renal failure
Hyaline	Nonspecific/oliguria
RBC	Glomerulonephritis
WBC	Glomerulonephritis
Epithelial	Nephrotic syndrome, acute tubular injury
Fatty	Nephrotic syndrome
Granular	Tubular injury
Bacteria	Infection
Crystals	Metabolic diseases

performed on all patients with a fever of unknown origin.

SERUM CHEMISTRIES

Analysis of serum encompasses a group of tests that are far beyond the scope of this text. The tests noted below are those that are most relevant to chiropractic practice. Some tests, although not a part of everyday general practice, have been included so that an overall picture of the patient's health can be formed.

The tests in this section are listed alphabetically. Normal values are noted parenthetically and the clinical significance of deviations from normal are also included.

Acid Phosphatase (<3 ng/mL or <0.8 IU/L)

This is a radioimmunoassay used in the evaluation of disease of the prostate gland.

Increase: (Metastatic) prostate cancer, prostatitis, benign prostatic hypertrophy

Alanine Aminotransaminase (ALT) (8–20 U/L)

See serum glutamic-pyruvic transaminase (SGPT).

Albumin (3.2–5.5 g/dL)

Albumin is protein measured for the evaluation of the kidneys and reticuloendothelial system as well as some connective tissue and gastrointestinal disorders. It is a relatively nonspecific test.

Decrease: Multiple myeloma, Hodgkin's disease, leukemia, renal disease (nephrotic syndrome), inflammatory bowel diseases, hepatic disease, collagen-vascular diseases

Albumin/Globulin Ratio (A/G Ratio) (1.0–2.2)

This is another relatively nonspecific test used in the evaluation of bone, liver, and renal diseases.

Decrease: Multiple myeloma, nephrotic syndrome, cirrhosis, and other hepatic disease

Alkaline Phosphatase (20–70 U/L)
(child = 20–40 IU/L)

This is an enzyme produced by both bone and liver tissue. Mildy elevated levels of this enzyme may be seen in children during adolescence and should not be mistaken for an abnormality. It may be necessary in some cases to fractionate the alkaline phosphatase to ascertain which organ system is causing the overproduction. Gamma-glutamyl transpeptidase determination is also helpful in making the distinction.

Increase: Bone malignancy, Paget's disease of bone, rickets/osteomalacia, hyperparathyroidism, hepatic disease, hyperthyroidism

Decrease: Excess vitamin D intake, malnutrition

Alpha-fetoprotein (AFP) (<25 ng/mL)

This is a serum study used in the evaluation of cancer and in the prenatal evaluation of the mother's serum for predicting spina bifida.

Increase: Hepatic carcinoma, testicular carcinoma, spina bifida

Amylase (25–125 U/L)

Amylase is an enzyme produced by the pancreas that causes the breakdown of complex sugars. Elevation is most often associated with disease of the pancreas.

Increase: Acute pancreatic disease, cholecystitis, peptic ulcer disease, mumps, renal disease, alcohol ingestion

Decrease: Pancreatic destruction, hepatic disease

Antinuclear Antibody (ANA) (negative)

The presence of antibodies against nuclei is a good indicator of collagen-vascular disorders.

Positive: Systemic lupus erythematosus (SLE), scleroderma (progressive systemic sclerosis), rheumatoid arthritis (RA), lupus syndromes (drug-induced)

Antistreptolysin-O Titre (ASO) (<165 units)

Increase: Infections (group-A hemolytic streptococcus), collagen-vascular disease (rheumatoid arthritis)

Aspartate Aminotransferase (AST)

See serum glutamic oxaloacetic transaminase.

Bicarbonate (22–28 mEq/L)

This base acts as a buffer in the acid-base balance system.

Increase: Respiratory acidosis, as compensation for metabolic acidosis, chronic obstructive pulmonary disease

Decrease: Respiratory alkalosis, as compensation for metabolic alkalosis, diabetic ketoacidosis, severe diarrhea, salicylates

Bilirubin (Total = <0.2–1.2 mg/dL, indirect = <1.1 mg/dL, direct = <0.3 mg/dL)

This is the bile pigment formed mainly by the breakdown of red blood cells. The direct form is conjugated with glucuronide and the indirect form is unconjugated.

Increase (total): Hemolysis, hepatobiliary disease, fasting

Increase (direct): Hepatitis, biliary obstruction, drug-induced cholestasis (estrogen), hepatic cancer

Increase (indirect): Gilbert's syndrome, hemolysis

Blood Urea Nitrogen (BUN) (7–25 mg/dL)

This chemistry is used in conjunction with creatinine in determining normal renal function.

Increase: Renal failure, pre/postrenal azotemia, gastrointestinal hemorrhage, drugs (aminoglycosides)

Decrease: Hepatic failure, pregnancy, nephrotic syndrome

Calcium (8.5–10.6 mg/dL)

Increase: Bone tumors, osteoporosis, Paget's disease, sarcoidosis, hyperparathyroidism, immobilization, hyperthyroidism, excess vitamin D

Decrease: Osteomalacia, rickets, renal failure, hypoparathyroidism

Chloride (95–110 mEq/L)

Increase: Diarrhea, renal disease

Decrease: Vomiting, diabetic ketoacidosis, renal disease

Cholesterol (120–200 mg/dL)

Increase: Hypercholesterolemia, diabetes mellitus, hyperlipoproteinemia, pregnancy

Decrease: Hepatic disease, steroid therapy, malnutrition, chronic anemia

Creatine Phosphokinase (CPK) (25–150 IU/L)

This enzyme has classically been used for the determination of myocardial damage. It is also elevated in a number of other diseases. Myocardial band (CPK-MB), muscle band (CPK-MM), and brain band (CPK-BB) have been identified and can be fractionated in order to determine which organ has been damaged.

Increase: Muscle damage (myocardial infarction, muscle trauma, rhabdomyolysis, polymyositis), cerebrovascular accident

Creatinine (0.7–1.4 mg/dL)

This test is the best serum determination of normal renal function. It is used in combination with blood urea nitrogen.

Increase: Renal failure, acromegaly, muscle disease
Decrease: Pregnancy

Fluorescent Treponemal Antibody Absorbed (FTA-ABS) (nonreactive)

Positive: Syphilis or other treponemal diseases

Gamma-glutamyl Transpeptidase (GGT) (0–45 U/L)

Increase: Hepatic disease, pancreatic disease

Globulins (1.5–3.8 g/dL)

Increase: Infection, leukemia, multiple myeloma, hepatic disease
Decrease: Renal disease, hypogammaglobulinemia

Glucose (70–115 mg/dL)

This test should be performed after the patient has fasted for 12 hours.

Increase: Diabetes mellitus, acromegaly, Cushing's syndrome, acute pancreatitis
Decrease: Pancreatic disease, hepatic disease hypoglycemia, oral hypoglycemic drugs

Human Chorionic Gonadotropin (HCG) (<3.0 mU/mL)

The beta subunit of HCG is used in the determination of pregnancy. Urine HCG can also be measured.

Increase: Pregnancy, testicular cancer, choriocarcinoma, molar pregnancy

Human Immunodeficiency Virus (HIV)

See human T-lymphocyte virus.

Human T-Lymphocyte Virus (HTLV) (negative)

Positive: Acquired immune deficiency syndrome

Iron (40–155 μg/dL)

Increase: Hemochromatosis, hemosiderosis, hemolysis
Decrease: Iron deficiency anemia, chronic disease, chronic infection

Iron Binding Capacity (Total) (TIBC)
(250–410 μg/dL)
Increase: Hemorrhage, iron deficiency anemia, oral contraceptive agents, hepatic disease
Decrease: Chronic disease, chronic infection, hepatic cirrhosis, renal disease, hemochromatosis

Lactate Dehydrogenase (LDH) (0–250 U/L)
This enzyme is a nonspecific indicator of inflammation. Isoenzymes can also be fractionated.
Increase: Myocardial infarction, hepatic disease, malignant tumors, hemolysis, pulmonary and renal embolism/infarction

Lipase (0.0–2.0 U/mL)
This enzyme, which breaks down fats, is an indicator of pancreatic disease.
Increase: Acute pancreatitis, pancreatic duct obstruction

Lupus Erythematosus Cell Preparation (LE Prep)
(none seen)
This test is becoming less useful than previously thought.
Positive: Systemic lupus erythematosus (SLE), rheumatoid arthritis, scleroderma, drug-induced lupus-like syndromes (procainamide)

Monospot (negative)
This quick test is a useful tool in the diagnosis of infectious mononucleosis.
Positive: Infectious mononucleosis, viral hepatitis, rheumatoid arthritis (false positive), leukemias, lymphomas

Parathyroid Hormone (PTH) (100–600 pg/mL)
Increase: Primary and secondary hyperparathyroidism
Decrease: Idiopathic hypercalcemia, other non-parathyroid causes of hypercalcemia

Phosphorus (2.5–4.5 mg/dL)
Increase: Hypoparathyroidism, secondary hyperparathyroidism, bone diseases, renal failure
Decrease: Hyperparathyroidism, alcoholism, diabetes mellitus, gout, diuretic therapy, vitamin D deficiency

Potassium (3.5–5.3 mEq/L)
Increase: Renal failure, Addison's disease, hemolysis, potassium-containing drugs
Decrease: Diuretic therapy, vomiting, diarrhea, renal disease

Protein Electrophoresis (Serum) (SPE) (variable)

Serum proteins are fractionated into five groups: albumin, alpha-1 globulin, alpha-2 globulin, beta globulin, and the gamma globulins (IgA, IgG, IgM, IgD, IgE). The classic "M spike" (elevated albumin and gamma globulins) (Figure 9-2) is seen with multiple myeloma. Gamma globulin elevation is seen with collagen-vascular diseases, infections, and leukemia.

Protein, Serum (6.0–8.5 g/dL)

Increase: Multiple myeloma, sarcoidosis, acute inflammation

Decrease: Malnutrition, Hodgkin's disease, leukemia, inflammatory bowel disorders

Rheumatoid Factor (RA Latex) (<1:40)

The RA latex titre can be used as an indicator of the activity of the disease.

Increase: Rheumatoid arthritis, systemic lupus erythematosus, syphilis

Serum Glutamic-oxaloacetic Transaminase (SGOT) (0–50 U/L)

See also aspartate aminotransaminase.

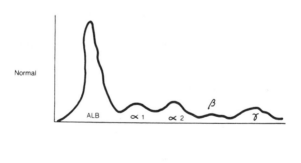

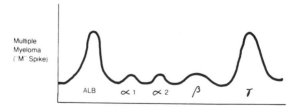

Figure 9-2 Serum Protein Electrophoresis Patterns

Increase: Hepatic disease, myocardial infarction, brain damage, renal disease, muscle disease

Serum Glutamic-pyruvic Transaminase (SGPT) (0–55 U/L)

See also alanine aminotransferase.

Increase: Hepatobiliary disease, pancreatitis

Sodium (135–148 mEq/L)

Increase: Cushing's syndrome, diabetes insipidus

Decrease: CHF, hepatic cirrhosis, renal failure, multiple myeloma, vomiting, diarrhea

Thyroid Stimulating Hormone (TSH) (0.5–5.0 μg/mL)

This test is good for screening for hypothyroidism.

Increase: Primary hypothyroidism

Decrease: Primary hyperthyroidism, pituitary insufficiency with secondary hypothyroidism

Thyroxine (T4 Total) (5–12 μg/dL)

This is an excellent screening test for hyperthyroidism.

Increase: Hyperthyroidism, pregnancy, estrogen therapy

Triglycerides (20–150 mg/dL)

Increase: Hyperlipoproteinemia, hepatic disease, alcoholism, renal disease, pancreatitis, myocardial infarction

Triiodothyronine (T3 RIA) (125–200 mg/dL)

Increase: Hyperthyroidism, pregnancy, estrogen therapy

Decrease: Hypothyroidism

Uric Acid (2.5–7.5 mg/dL)

Increase: Gout, renal failure, leukemia

Venereal Disease Research Laboratory (VDRL) (nonreactive)

This is a good screening test for syphilis that, if reactive, can be confirmed with FTA-ABS testing.

Positive: Syphilis, systemic lupus erythematosus (SLE) (false positive), pregnancy (false positive)

SPECIAL STUDIES

- *Erythrocyte Sedimentation Rate*—Elevation is a nonspecific indicator of inflammation somewhere in the body.

- *C-Reactive Protein*—Positive test is a nonspecific indicator of inflammation.
- *Hemoccult*—Used to diagnosis occult blood in the stool. For this test to be positive it must reveal occult blood on at least three separate occasions.

SPECIFIC LABORATORY PANELS

The investigation of specific organ system disease is augmented by the use of groups of laboratory tests specific to an organ or system. Exhibit 9-1 lists some of

Exhibit 9-1 Laboratory Profiles

Bone tumor profile
   Calcium
   Phosphorus
   Alkaline phosphatase
   Acid phosphatase (if blastic)
Arthritis profile
   RA latex
   Uric acid
   HLA-B27
   ESR
Kidney profile
   BUN
   Creatinine
   Albumin
   Globulin
   A/G ratio
Cardiac risk profile
   Cholesterol
   Triglycerides
   Glucose
Cardiac ischemia profile
   CPK-MB
   SGOT
   LDH
Hepatic profile
   SGPT
   SGOT
   LDH
   Bilirubin
   Albumin
   Globulin

the more common panels useful to the chiropractic clinician.

BIBLIOGRAPHY

Gomella, L., ed. 1989. *Clinician's pocket reference*. Norwalk, Conn.: Appleton & Lange.

Larson, E.B., and M.S. Eisenberg. 1987. *Manual of admitting orders and therapeutics*. Philadelphia: Harcourt Brace Jovanovich.

Wallach, J. 1978. *Interpretation of diagnostic tests: A handbook synopsis of laboratory medicine*. Boston: Little, Brown & Co.

10

Diagnostic Imaging

INTRODUCTION

Since its discovery, imaging of the human body has been a mainstay in the investigation of patient complaints. However, ionizing radiation is not without hazard. Its most deleterious effects are on body systems with the highest cell turnover such as the reproductive organs, the retinal and hematopoietic systems, and the gastrointestinal tract. It is for this reason that radiation in any form must be justified before use.

This chapter outlines the proper application of radiation in chiropractic. Much emphasis is placed on basic rules of radiology. If the basics are understood, it is much easier to accomplish the more in-depth aspects of clinical imaging. Protocols are also delineated.

There are ten basic rules of radiology that, when followed meticulously, will lead the clinician to the proper imaging study and an accurate diagnosis:

1. Consult often with a chiropractic radiologist. As a specialty consultant, the chiropractic radiologist can supply the physician with written reports to help with workers' compensation and personal injury claims. If there is ever a question regarding a radiographic finding or which study should be performed next, the chiropractic radiologist is very helpful.

2. Perform only those studies that are clinically justified. Ask this simple question: "Will the treatment or the prognosis for the patient change if this study is performed?" If the answer is yes, then the study should be performed, barring any contraindications. If the answer is no, then serious thought should be given to other diagnostic studies that might be more helpful.

3. Choose the correct imaging procedure. If a patient presents with elbow pain that, after history and physical examination, appears to result from intrinsic elbow disease, x-ray the elbow. Radiating the cervical spine, shoulder, or wrist, if one of them is not the cause of the complaint, is often unjustified. If a patient has signs of spinal cord disease, then a magnetic resonance imaging (MRI) scan is the proper procedure, not a computerized tomography (CT) scan. Selection of the proper procedure yields the clinician the most valuable information possible.

4. Always perform a complete series. This includes a minimum of 90-degree views of the area of chief complaint. If there is clinical suspicion that a patient may have true radiculopathy from cervical foraminal encroachment, then oblique views of the cervical spine are in order.

5. Establish a standard protocol for working in the radiography suite; this insures that a marker is never left off, for example.

6. Accept only good quality radiographs. It is a disservice to both the clinician and the patient to accept anything less. Poor quality films serve no useful purpose and even may result in a malpractice suit. It is certainly worth the added effort necessary to achieve quality.

7. Develop a pattern approach to radiographic interpretation. If a pattern is established while viewing radiographs, the pattern soon becomes a routine and it becomes less likely that subtle but ominous radiographic signs will be missed.

8. Compare with previous films, if at all possible. There is no better way to assess a patient's progress or poor response than with serial radiography although reradiography in patients with biomechanical, nonpathological spine pain is most often fruitless. For example, a pulmonary

nodule that remains unchanged after 2 years is almost certainly benign. Without comparison films, the patient may have to undergo painful and expensive procedures to rule out a malignant lesion.

9. Understand the basic tenets of radiographic interpretation. There are several rules, germane to all radiographic studies, that should be rigidly followed. Utilization of these rules, which are presented in the next section, will help prevent oversight of any serious pathology.

10. Always have a written report in the patient's chart. Maintenance of a written report along with the views performed and the factors used to expose the patient are an integral part of any patient file.

BASIC RULES OF RADIOGRAPHIC INTERPRETATION

There are a number of basic rules in radiology that should be memorized, understood, and utilized any time the clinician interprets a radiographic study. The following are only guidelines; there are exceptions to these rules but, in most instances, the rules will be helpful.

General Bone Radiology

1. Osteopenia is a radiographic description of loss of bone density; osteoporosis is a disease. The diagnosis of osteoporosis can seldom be made from a radiograph. Clinical signs and symptoms should be consistent with the diagnosis.

2. Hyperemia causes osteopenia; avascular necrosis causes osteosclerosis.

3. Painful lesions are usually aggressive; nonpainful lesions are usually benign.

4. Slow growing lesions are usually nonaggressive.

Bone Tumors

1. A solitary lytic/blastic lesion in a patient over 40 is malignant until proven otherwise; consider metastasis and multiple myeloma.

2. A solitary diaphyseal lucency in any patient is malignant until proven otherwise; consider leukemia and metastatic neuroblastoma in children and reticuloendothelial malignancies in adults.
3. The most common skeletal malignancy is lytic metastasis. Table 10-1 outlines the most common sites of primary malignancies that metastasize to the skeleton.
4. Symmetry suggests a normal variant.
5. Patients over 40 years of age have malignancies; patients under 40 have benign lesions.
6. Diffuse osteopenia in a male may be the only sign of multiple myeloma.
7. Calcified lesions are usually benign (except chondrosarcoma).
8. Thick sclerosis around the edge of a lesion suggests benignancy; consider fibrous lesions.
9. Thirty to fifty percent bone destruction is required before any plain film radiographic findings become evident.
10. Metastasis favors the pedicles; multiple myeloma spares the pedicles.
11. Long lesions in long bones usually have a fibrous matrix.

Arthritides

1. Older patients have degenerative arthritides; younger patients have inflammatory arthritides.
2. Always rule out atlantoaxial instability in any patient with inflammatory arthritis; consider transverse ligament rupture.

Table 10-1 Primary Cancers That Metastasize to Bone and Their Most Common Radiographic Appearances

Location of Cancer	Radiographic Appearance
Breast	lytic
	blastic
	mixed
Lung	lytic
Thyroid	lytic
Kidney	lytic
Prostate	blastic

3. Bilateral symmetry suggests rheumatoid arthritis.
4. Inflammatory arthritis in young males is most often due to a seronegative spondyloarthropathy; consider ankylosing spondylitis.
5. A monarticular arthritis is infectious until proven otherwise.
6. Pure bone erosion without bone production suggests rheumatoid arthritis; bone erosion with bone production suggests a seronegative spondyloarthropathy.
7. Degenerative joint disease is, by far, the most common form of arthritis.
8. Degenerative joint disease in an articulation that does not normally develop degenerative joint disease is probably secondary to crystal deposition or trauma.

Trauma

1. Compression fractures where both the anterior and posterior vertebral body heights are lost are pathologic until proven otherwise.
2. Transverse fractures are pathologic until proven otherwise.
3. Avulsion of the lesser trochanter is pathologic until proven otherwise.
4. Multiple injuries at different stages of healing indicate battered child syndrome (child abuse) until proven otherwise.
5. Spiral fractures in children are suspicious for child abuse.
6. Metaphyseal beak fractures are almost pathognomonic for child abuse.
7. Symmetry suggests a normal variant; consider nonfusion of a secondary growth center. Do comparison views when necessary.
8. Distraction and rotation of fracture fragments are ominous prognostic indicators.
9. A healed fracture is a clinical decision, not a radiographic one.
10. If there is a greater than 25% compression of vertebral body height, order a CT scan to rule out retropulsion of bone fragments into the spinal canal.

Infection

1. Rapid progression of a lesion, days to weeks, usually suggests an infectious etiology.
2. Infections invade and blur fascial planes; tumors deflect fascial planes.
3. Joints are especially vulnerable to tuberculosis.
4. Multifocal infections are found in infants and geriatric patients.
5. Infection, along with infarction and avascular necrosis, suggests sickle cell anemia.

Congenital Lesions

1. If there is one anomaly, look for another.
2. Lumbosacral transitional segments are best not called sacralization or lumbarization.
3. Lumbar spine anomalies are often associated with genitourinary anomalies.

Soft Tissues

Abdomen

Although most chiropractic practices concentrate on bone and joint radiology, there are many times when evaluation of soft tissues with radiography becomes necessary, as noted below.

1. The maximum normal anteroposterior diameter of the abdominal aorta is 3.5 centimeters. Anything larger suggests an abdominal aortic aneurysm.
2. The most common abdominal calcification is a calcified mesenteric lymph node.
3. The most common pelvic calcification occurs in the pelvic veins (phlebolith).
4. Absence or haziness of a fascial plane suggests inflammation (peritonitis).
5. The maximum normal diameters of the small and large intestines are 3.0 and 5.0 centimeters, respectively. Significant enlargement suggests obstruction or adynamic ileus.

Chest

1. The cardiac silhouette should be no larger than one-half the largest lateral measurement of the thoracic cage.
2. The first diagnostic step after finding a pulmonary mass is to compare the most recent film with previous films. Growth of the lesion during a 2-year period should be looked upon with suspicion for malignancy, while stability for 2 years suggests benignancy.
3. Chest films with a less than full inspiration give the false appearance of congestive heart failure.
4. Deviation of the trachea suggests that either something is pushing it away (mass) or pulling it towards (atelectasis) the side of the lesion.
5. Calcification within a pulmonary lesion, especially when centrally located, suggests benignancy.

DIFFERENTIAL DIAGNOSIS AND FOLLOW-UP IMAGING

One of the most challenging aspects of radiology is to determine, once the lesion is located, what the next step is for the patient. Table 10-2 outlines the differential diagnosis of common radiographic signs and the procedures of choice for further workup.

Patient Referral

Many times, it becomes prudent for patients with aggressive lesions to be referred to another physician for diagnosis or treatment. To determine if such referral is necessary, characterize the lesion using the information in Exhibits 10-1, 10-2, and 10-3 and Table 10-3.

Common Causes of Common Lesions

Table 10-4 lists the most common causes of some common lesions.

Table 10-2 Differential Diagnosis and Follow-up Imaging for Lesions

Diagnosis	Radiographic Sign	Additional Procedure
Blastic Lesion (solitary)	Metastasis	Positive bone scan
	Bone island	Painless—negative bone scan
	Osteoid osteoma	Nidus—positive bone scan
	Stress fracture	History—positive bone scan
Blastic Lesions (multiple)	Metastasis	Positive bone scan
	Osteopoikilosis	Painless—negative bone scan
Chondrocalcinosis*	Idiopathic Degenerative joint disease Calcium pyrophosphate crystal deposition disease Gouty arthritis (soft tissue masses, hyperuricemia)	
Lucent Lesion (solitary)	Metastasis	Positive bone scan
	Multiple myeloma	Negative bone scan, serum protein electrophoresis (SPE)
	Benign tumor	Young patient; +/− bone scan; +/− pain
Lucent Lesions (multiple)	Metastasis	Positive bone scan
	Multiple myeloma	Negative bone scan, SPE
Missing Pedicle	Metastasis	Positive bone scan

*Joint aspiration is the only way to make a definitive diagnosis.

continues

Table 10-2 continued

Diagnosis	Radiographic Sign	Additional Procedure
	Agenesis	Contralateral pedicle sclerosis
Multiloculated Lesion	Aneurysmal bone cyst	Painful, posttraumatic
	Chondroblastoma	Epiphyseal/ apophyseal
	Enchondroma	Hands; painless
	Fibrous dysplasia	Thick sclerotic rim
	Giant cell tumor	Subarticular location
	Hemangioma	Striated appearance; painless
	Nonossifying fibroma	Adolescent, eccentric, sclerosis
	Osteoblastoma	Painful, spine/ neural arch
	Plasmacytoma	Painful, SPE
	Solitary bone cyst	Painless, proximal humerus/femur
Osteopenia in a Male	Multiple myeloma	Negative bone scan, SPE
	Metastasis	Positive bone scan
	Osteoporosis	Negative bone scan, negative SPE
Sacroilitis	Ankylosing spondylitis	Male, bilateral symmetry
	Other seronegative spondyloarthrop-athies	Asymmetry
	Infection	Unilateral
Sclerotic Vertebrae	Metastasis	Positive bone scan, no change in size
	Paget's disease	Enlarged, hypertrabeculat-ed, thick cortex
	Lymphoma	Anterior body scalloping
	Idiopathic	Exclusion of all others

Exhibit 10-1 Benign Lesions of Bone

Signs of Benignancy

Small size
Thick rim of sclerosis
Thick or no periosteal reaction
Cortical expansion without destruction
No soft tissue mass
Geographic pattern of bone destruction
Calcification (except for chondrosarcoma)
Negative bone scan

Types of Benign Bone Lesions

Cartilaginous
   Enchondroma
   Osteochondroma
   Chondroblastoma
Osseous
   Enostoma (bone island)
   Osteoma
   Osteoblastoma
Fibrous
   Fibroxanthoma
   Fibrous dysplasia

RADIATION PHYSICS MADE EASY

The following basic rules help make radiation physics more easily understood, especially as far as applying physics to everyday clinical practice.

1. Milliampere-seconds (mAs) control density (blackness) of the radiograph. The relationship of this setting to density is generally linear, i.e., doubling the mAs will cause a doubling of film blackness. Use mAs and not kilovoltage potential to control density. There must be at least a 30% change in mAs for a change to be seen on the radiograph. Change the mAs by changing the time, not the mA.

2. Kilovoltage potential (kVp) controls contrast (number of shades of grey). Its relationship to film density is logarithmic. Do not use kVp to control density. The only time to vary kVp from standard protocols (depicted in Figure 10-1) is with obese patients. Use lower kVp to reduce

Exhibit 10-2 Aggressive Lesions of Bone

Signs of Aggressiveness

Large size
Absence of sclerotic rim
Laminated or spiculated periosteal reaction
Cortical destruction
Soft tissue mass
Moth-eaten or permeative bone destruction
No calcification (except for chondrosarcoma)
Positive bone scan

Types of Aggressive Bone Lesions

Osteomyelitis
Cartilaginous
  Chondrosarcoma
Osseous
  Osteosarcoma
Fibrous
  Fibrosarcoma
Miscellaneous
  Multiple myeloma
  Giant cell tumor

scatter radiation and thus reduce film fog. If the patient measures over 30 centimeters, a general rule is to increase kVp by 2 for each centimeter over 30. If the outlines of the bones can be seen, enough kVp has been used. Film density can now be controlled with mAs.

3. Any body part measuring over 13 centimeters should be x-rayed with a grid to reduce scatter radiation.

4. Always err on the side of too much density. An underexposed film is useless, unless of course a foreign body in the soft tissues is being sought.

5. Always use the shortest time and longest patient-to-film distance possible to reduce magnification, distortion, and patient motion.

6. The inverse square law is useful if the clinician moves the tube (e.g. from 40 inches to 72 inches for a lateral lumbar spine film).

Exhibit 10-3 Unstable Lesions of Bone

Signs of Instability

Vertebral body compression of more than 25%
Anterolisthesis of more than 25% of vertebra below
Sagittal rotation of more than 11 degrees
Atlantodental interspace of greater than
    5 mm in children
    3 mm in adults
Retropulsion of bone fragments into spinal canal

Types of Unstable Bone Lesions

Cervical spine
    Odontoid fractures (Types II and III)
    Flexion teardrop fracture
    Extension teardrop fracture
    Burst fracture
    Bilateral facet dislocation
Thoracolumbar spine
    Burst fracture
    Bilateral facet dislocation
    Chance fracture

Radiology Reports

Radiology reports should adhere to the following format:

- name, age, and sex of the patient
- studies performed
- date of the study and report
- body of the report (paragraph form)

Table 10-3 Patterns of Bone Destruction

Pattern	Description	Significance
Geographic	Large, well defined	Benign
Moth-eaten	Mid-sized, ill defined	Aggressive
Permeative	Pinpoint, ill defined	Aggressive

Table 10-4 Common Causes of Common Lesions

Lesion	Cause
Bone tumors	
Skeletal malignancy	Lytic metastasis
Primary skeletal malignancy	Multiple myeloma
Tumor to metastasize to skeleton	Bronchogenic carcinoma
Benign tumor of skeleton	Bone island (enostoma)
Benign tumor of spine	Hemangioma
Diffuse osteopenia	Osteoporosis
Arthritides	
Arthritis	Degenerative joint disease (DJD)
Destructive arthritis	Rheumatoid arthritis
Lumps and bumps around joints	DJD
Skeletal trauma	
Fracture plane in adults	Oblique
Fractured bone in body	Clavicle
Fracture of spine	Simple compression fracture
Fractured bone in wrist	Scaphoid
Fracture of elbow	Radial head
Fracture of hip	Subcapital
Dislocation of shoulder	Anteroinferior
Dislocated bone in wrist	Lunate
Dislocation of hip	Posterior
Location of osteochondritis dissecans	Medial femoral condyle

- impressions (conclusions from the body)
- comments (recommendations for further investigation)
- signature

To increase clarity and readability, follow these guidelines in writing reports:

1. Be brief without forsaking completeness. Include only the pertinent positives and pertinent negatives.
2. Write in a narrative format and use short, complete sentences.
3. Use the present tense when referring to what is seen on the film. Use the past tense only when referring to previous studies.

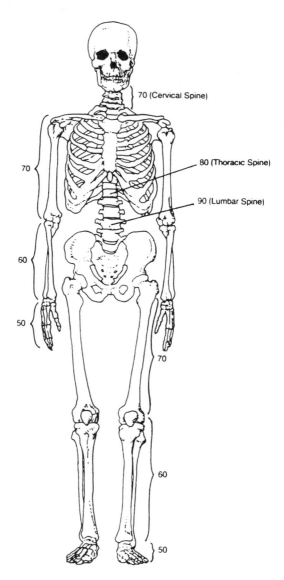

Figure 10-1 Standard KVP for Different Body Regions

4. Avoid using phrases like "there is" at the beginning of sentences. It becomes monotonous to the reader.
5. If there is a specific question regarding, for example, trauma, explain that "no fractures are identified" in the report.

6. Vary the wording of reports. Using the same sentences consistently runs the risk of missing an important but subtle finding.
7. Note the most important findings first and save the incidentals for last.
8. Save diagnostic conclusions for the impressions section of the report.
9. Clearly express any clinical impressions and the confidence felt in each.

Advanced Diagnostic Imaging

Use of advanced imaging has become common in the modern chiropractic practice. These modalities can be helpful in the diagnostic, treatment, and prognostic decisions that must be made regarding patient care.

Computerized Tomography (CT)

Computerized axial tomography, while utilizing x-radiation as an imaging source, can be extremely helpful in diagnosing many osseous and soft tissue lesions. While much controversy exists regarding the utility of CT in the diagnosis of central nervous system disease, especially with the advent of magnetic resonance imaging, it is still useful in a number of different instances (see Exhibit 10-4).

Patients who will require iodinated contrast agents during a CT examination should be queried regarding any allergy or adverse reaction to iodine.

Magnetic Resonance Imaging (MRI)

MRI has become a staple in the investigation of central nervous system disorders in recent years. It has also become popular in the evaluation of patients with suspected disc disease. It does not require the use of ionizing radiation and has very few side effects. Exhibit 10-5 outlines the indications and contraindications for using MRI.

Radionuclide Bone Scanning

The chiropractic doctor is often called upon to evaluate the possibility of malignancy in a patient. The intravenous injection of a radiopharmaceutical that has an affinity for bone (i.e., bone scanning) is a help-

Exhibit 10-4 Common Indications for Computerized Tomography

Motor vehicle accidents
Follow-up of unusual plain film findings
- Clinically significant subluxation
- Spinal canal/foraminal stenosis
- Fractures/dislocations
- Clinically significant congenital anomalies
- Infection
- Tumor

Abdominal masses (e.g., abdominal aortic aneurysm)
Herniated nucleus pulposus
Intracanalicular space-occupying lesions
Headache of unknown etiology
Cauda equina syndrome
Cerebral space-occupying lesions
Postoperative pain
Cerebral ischemia

ful procedure in this task. A gamma camera is used to detect any areas in the skeleton that uptake an abnormal amount of the radiotracer. Exhibit 10-6 outlines the more common indications for radionuclide bone scans.

Diagnostic Ultrasound (US)

The use of sound waves has become useful in the diagnosis of soft tissue diseases of the human body.

Exhibit 10-5 When To Use Magnetic Resonance Imaging

Common Indications

Central nervous system disease
Disc disease
Spinal canal stenosis
Arnold-Chiari malformation
Spinal trauma

Contraindications

Pregnancy
Cerebral aneurysm clips
Cardiac pacemaker

Exhibit 10-6 Common Indications for Bone Scanning

Skeletal metastasis
Primary bone tumors
Osteomyelitis

Exhibit 10-7 Common Indications for Diagnostic Ultrasound

Pregnancy
Uterine disease
Ovarian disease
Gallbladder disease
Abdominal aortic aneurysm

US has become most popular in the evaluation of abdominal and pelvic organs. It also shows promise in the investigation of musculoskeletal diseases. Exhibit 10-7 demonstrates some of the indications for diagnostic US for the chiropractic patient.

BIBLIOGRAPHY

Chew, F. 1990. *Skeletal radiology: The bare bones.* Gaithersburg, Md.: Aspen Publishers, Inc.

Daffner, R. 1988. *Imaging of vertebral trauma.* Gaithersburg, Md.: Aspen Publishers, Inc.

Jaeger, S., and D. Pate. 1990. *Case studies in chiropractic radiology.* Gaithersburg, Md.: Aspen Publishers, Inc.

Juhl, L., and A. Crummy. 1987. *Essentials of radiologic imaging.* Philadelphia: J.B. Lippincott.

Yochum, T., and L. Rowe. 1987. *Essentials of skeletal radiology.* Baltimore: Williams & Wilkins Co.

11

Procedures Used in Clinical Practice

INTRODUCTION

This chapter outlines the many procedures that are germane to and used in chiropractic practice. No attempt has been made to justify the procedures or their rationale. Instead, the proper steps taken for each procedure are included. The bibliography at the end of this chapter gives sources of further information.

Venipuncture (Phlebotomy)

Definition: The insertion of a needle into a peripheral vein so that venous blood can be withdrawn for analysis.

Materials

- Tourniquet
- Alcohol pad
- Specimen tubes (see Table 11-1)

Table 11-1 Blood Specimen Tubes

Tube	Test(s)
Red top	Serum studies
Purple top	Complete blood count
Green top	HLA-B27
Grey top	Glucose tolerance test
Tiger top	Serum studies
Royal blue top	Heavy metals

- An 18–22 gauge needle (the smaller the gauge the larger the needle)
- Vacutainer holder
- Gauze/cotton balls
- Bandaids

Procedure

1. Have all the necessary materials close at hand and easily accessible.
2. Palpate the antecubital fossa for prominent veins (Figure 11-1) and select the one to be used. To make the veins more easily visible/palpable, have the patient pump the hand by opening and closing the fist; then gently but briskly tap on the fossa with your index and middle fingers.
3. Apply the tourniquet approximately 5 to 10 cms above the site of puncture. Then have the patient make a fist and hold it. Relocate the vein to be used and follow its course for a short distance proximally.
4. Swab the area with the alcohol prep. Wipe off any excess alcohol with gauze or cotton.

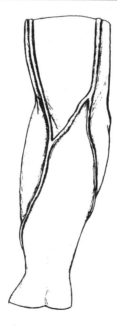

Figure 11-1 Veins of the Right Antecubital Fossa

5. Insert the needle and tube into the holder in their proper respective positions but do not puncture the rubber stopper on the tube yet.
6. Insert the needle with the bevel up (Figure 11-2) into the skin adjacent to the vein. After the needle is through the skin, stabilize the vein with your free hand to prevent it from rolling.
7. Enter the vein at approximately a 30° angle, being careful not to pierce through the opposite side of the vein.
8. Withdraw the sample by piercing the rubber stopper on the tube with the needle in the holder by advancing the tube forward. The vacuum inside the tube will automatically collect the sample.
9. If another tube is to be drawn, gently remove the first tube from the holder, place it aside, and insert the new tube onto the needle. Repeat this same procedure for any other tubes that need to be drawn.
10. After the sample(s) have been drawn, remove the tourniquet, withdraw the needle, and apply firm pressure on the puncture site with a small

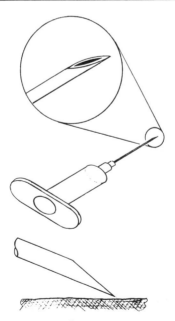

Note: The bevel of the needle is up.

Figure 11-2 Proper Needle Insertion for Venipuncture

piece of gauze folded into quarters. Elevating the extremity may be helpful.
11. Place tape over the folded gauze and assure that the patient tolerated the procedure well.
12. Perform whatever procedures are necessary for preparation of the sample for study, such as centrifugation.

Urine Specimen Collection

Definition: Collection of a patient's urine so that urine can be analyzed for the presence of a number of different chemicals, cells, and crystals.

Materials

• Urine collection cup and label

Procedure (for clean catch specimen)

1. Instruct the patient to go into the bathroom and to follow the procedures listed below.
   • Have the patient void a small amount of urine and then stop the stream. This purges the urethra of any residual sediment.
   • The patient should begin the stream again and urinate into the container provided until the cup is half full, and then void the remaining urine. If the patient cannot fill the cup half full, have him or her void until the bladder is almost empty and then stop the stream.
2. The specimen should be examined immediately, as urine degrades rather quickly in warm temperatures. If some time will elapse before the specimen will be examined, it should be refrigerated.

Vertebrobasilar/Carotid Artery Testing

Definition: Testing the vertebrobasilar arterial system for patency to prevent any ischemic event during manipulation. This should be performed on all patients undergoing cervical spine manipulation, as often as is deemed clinically necessary. For example, patients with previous positive findings or those at high risk for stroke should have testing performed more often than those at very low risk. At the very least, testing should be performed during the initial physical examination.

Materials

- Stethoscope

Procedure

1. The patient should be seated comfortably.
2. The doctor should face the patient and carefully palpate the carotid artery on the right and then the carotid artery on the left. The arteries should never be palpated simultaneously. Bilateral palpation may induce bradycardia and possible syncope, especially in the older patient.
3. The carotid arteries should then be auscultated with the bell of the stethoscope. A search should be made for bruits, which are a sign of arterial stenosis or aneurysm. Any abnormal sounds should be noted.
4. Auscultation of the subclavian arteries (in the supraclavicular fossae) and regions of the vertebral arteries should then be performed. Again, any adventitious sounds are noted.
5. The skull should then be auscultated (with the bell of the stethoscope) for bruits and the findings duly registered.
6. Using the bell of the stethoscope, the orbital regions are auscultated for abnormal sounds, such as bruits.
7. The patient's head is first fully extended and rotated and held in that position for 60 seconds. A search is made for nystagmus and the patient is questioned concerning dizziness or vertigo.
8. The same procedure is then followed with the patient's head fully flexed and rotated. The same questions are asked.

Notes: Any abnormal findings demonstrated in these tests are noted. The risks versus benefits of manipulation on each particular patient are then considered. In general, positive findings are relative contraindications for aggressive manipulation of the cervical spine. Rotary forms of adjusting are the most commonly implicated factor in complications from cervical spine manipulation.

Electrocardiogram (ECG, EKG)

Definition: Measuring the electrical conducting system of the heart to diagnose disease of the heart and other organ systems.

Materials

- Electrocardiographic machine with electrodes
- Electrode gel or prefabricated electrode pads.

(Machines used for ECGs vary with the institution. Some are even automated. Become familiar with the specific machine used in a specific institution.)

Procedure

1. Be certain the patient is comfortably positioned in the supine position.
2. Explain the procedure to the patient and assure him or her that there is no pain involved. Also insure that the patient understands the importance of remaining motionless during the examination. This will prevent any artifacts that would obscure proper interpretation of the examination.
3. Plug in the ECG machine and turn it on.
4. Attach each of the electrodes as outlined below (also see Figure 11-3)
   - Most often the color coding system delineates the proper placement of the electrodes.
     White—right arm (RA)

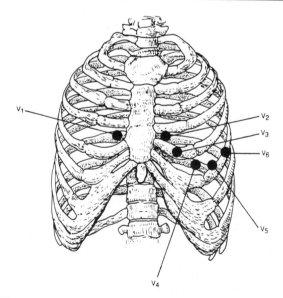

Figure 11-3 Proper ECG Electrode Placement

Black—left arm (LA)
Green—right leg (RL)
Red—left leg (LL)
Brown—chest ($V_1, V_2, V_3, V_4, V_5, V_6$)

- Each of the limb leads is attached along the distal ventral portion of the extremity. Apply electrode gel unless premoistened electrode pads are available.

- The placement of the precordial leads is as follows:
  V_1—Fourth ICS to the right of the sternum
  V_2—Fourth ICS to the left of the sternum
  V_3—Midway between leads V_2 and V_4
  V_4—Midclavicular line above the left fifth ICS
  V_5—Left fifth ICS at the anterior axillary line
  V_6—Left fifth ICS at midaxillary line

5. Once the leads are in proper position and the machine is ready, follow the instructions for that particular machine and obtain the tracings.
6. Label the tracing with the patient's name and age, the date and time, and both your and the attending physician's names.

Radiography
Definition: Using ionizing radiation and plain film examination to investigate pathology.
Materials

- X-ray unit
- X-ray film
- Positioning aids (if necessary)
- X-ray technique calculator
- Film processor
- Right/left side markers
- Filters
- Gonad shields
- Lead gloves/apron
- Measuring calipers

Procedure: Although x-ray units and positioning for each radiographic view differ, the same procedure can be used on all patients to ensure excellent radiographs in all cases. (These procedures are also summarized in Exhibit 11-1).

Exhibit 11-1 Radiography Procedures

```
Explain procedure to patient
Insure the ten day rule applies
Obtain informed consent
Have patient undress and don gown
Remove jewelry
Measure part to be x-rayed
Input technique factors
Insert cassette with marker
Position the patient
Check focal film distance
Tilt tube
Position central ray
Recheck positioning
Give breathing instructions
Make the exposure
```

1. Explain the procedure, including the benefits and risks, to the patient. If the patient is a female, ensure that the procedure is being performed within 10 days after the onset of her last menstrual period. This rule applies unless the health of the mother is in imminent danger.

2. Obtain the informed consent of the patient for the x-ray procedures to be performed. Have a witness sign the form.

3. Have the patient undress and don a gown. Make certain the patient has removed any clothing or jewelry which may contain metal (earrings, brassieres, etc.).

4. Measure the body part to be examined with calipers.

5. Input the measurement into the technique chart or the technique calculator and figure the proper radiographic exposure factors. Always remember to use the shortest time possible.

6. Input the technique factors into the x-ray machine.

7. Place the x-ray cassette with the side marker attached into the tray or on the tabletop, whichever is necessary for the view being performed. Ensure the film tray is pushed all the way into the bucky.

8. Position the patient properly, including any rotation or tilting necessary.

9. Tilt the x-ray tube as necessary. Remember that tube tilt must be compensated for by decreasing the tube film distance 1 inch for every 5 degrees of tube tilt.
10. Place the central ray in the proper position, making sure it is centered with the film in the holder or on the tabletop.
11. Recheck all positioning and insure the proper factors have been programmed into the machine.
12. Give the patient the proper breathing instructions.
13. Expose the patient, ensuring that the button(s) is (are) depressed until the "beep" is heard.

Rectal Examination
Definition: Digital examination of the rectum and prostate for any palpable signs of pathology. Many rectal polyps can be found with digital examination. Because of the frequency of colon carcinoma, digital examination of the rectum and testing for occult blood should be performed on patients over 40. It should be remembered that this procedure is uncomfortable and many times embarrassing for patients. Reassuring the patient and explaining the procedure as it is being performed will help allay some of those fears.
Materials

- Lubricating gel
- Examination glove or finger cot
- Occult blood testing materials

Procedure: There are a number of different positions that can be used for proper examination of the patient. Use the one that will be most comfortable for the patient and most useful for the physician. The positions are listed below:

- *Left lateral decubitus*—Best position when evaluating for rectal masses. The patient lies on the left side with the knees pulled up comfortably up to the chest.
- *Knee-chest position*—Best position for palpating the prostate. The patient is placed on the table on his knees with his head and shoulders touching the examining table.

- *Dorsolithotomy position*—Particularly useful when examining female patients.
- *Bent over a table*—Useful for examining the prostate. The table should be waist high for patient comfort.

1. Position the patient.
2. The anal region should be inspected for signs of pathology such as hemorrhoids, fissures, fistulae, and skin lesions. Any pain or tenderness should be noted.
3. Place a small amount of lubricant on the index finger of the gloved hand.
4. Apply gentle but steady pressure on the anal sphincter while having the patient perform a Valsalva maneuver. This will facilitate entry.
5. Palpate the walls of the rectum for any signs of a mass or tenderness.
6. If the patient is a male, the finger is then rotated until the prostate gland is felt. It is then plapated for size, consistency, masses, and tenderness. Any masses are noted as to their size, tenderness, consistency, and contour. The normal prostate is a bi-lobed, nontender, smooth midline structure about the size of a walnut. Normal prostatic tissue feels similar to the feel of the tip of the nose.
7. Have the patient bear down again. This may make lesions that were beyond reach palpable.
8. The finger is gently withdrawn and the character of the stool on the gloved finger is noted. Black tarry stool is consistent with proximal GI tract bleeding. This stool is then checked for occult blood. (Standard tests for occult blood are available in most laboratories.)

Breast Examination

Definition: Visual and palpatory examination of the breast for the detection of pathology. This examination is no longer reserved for females, as the incidence of breast carcinoma in males has increased substantially. As the physician is performing the examination, he or she can explain the procedure to the patient. The patient can then repeat the examination for the doctor and then periodically perform the procedure at home, the best time being just after the cessation of menses. Breast self-examination is essential in the early detection of breast cancer.

Materials

- Mirror
- Good lighting

Procedure

1. Explain the procedure to the patient and ask him or her to indicate if there is any tenderness during any part of the procedure.
2. Have the patient sit, disrobe to the waist, and dangle arms at side.
3. Inspect the breasts for size, symmetry, and contour. Small variations in size are common but any dimpling or flattening of the skin or the visualization of masses must be noted. The color and venous patterns as well as edema or thickening of the skin should be noted. Any change in the nipples, including rashes, ulcerations, and discharge, are charted.
4. Perform the same visual inspection two more times, once with the patient's arms raised above the head and once with the hands down against the hips. The patient should also lean over so that a search for any adhesions can be made.
5. Each breast is then palpated by using three fingers of the hand and moving the fingers in a circular motion while moving centrifugally around the breast. Special attention should be paid to the upper outer quadrant of the breast, as this is the most common location for masses. Any nodules or masses should be palpated for location, size, consistency, shape, mobility, and tenderness. A large, nontender, nonmobile hard mass suggests cancer. The axilla is then palpated for any signs of nodules or masses; the same characteristics should be sought. The nipple is then gently squeezed for any signs of discharge. (Signs of breast cancer are listed in Exhibit 11-2.)
6. The same procedure is then performed with the patient in the supine position.

Cardiopulmonary Resuscitation (CPR)

Definition: The administration of external cardiac compressions and breathing to sustain a clinically dead patient until advanced cardiac life support can be initiated. The procedures used here are based on the

Exhibit 11-2 Signs of Breast Cancer

Breast lump/mass
Nipple discharge
Skin dimpling
"Orange peel" skin
Ulceration
Focal hypervascularity

Standards and Guidelines for Cardiopulmonary Resuscitation and Emergency Cardiac Care from the *Journal of the American Medical Association* (volume 255, number 21, 1986).

Materials: No special materials are necessary.

Procedures: CPR is most easily remembered by using the mnemonic ABC: airway, breathing, and circulation. It is assumed that the reader has been trained in CPR; the procedure noted here is in quick reference form. Remember that even with the best CPR technique, one is delivering only approximately one-third of normal cardiac output.

Adult CPR

1. Assess the level of responsiveness of the patient by shaking and shouting at patient.
2. If the patient is unresponsive, call loudly for help.
3. Place the patient in the supine position on a flat firm surface. If the patient is in a bed or on an adjusting table move him or her to the floor.
4. Ascertain whether the patient has spontaneous respirations. Tilt the patient's head using the head tilt-chin lift maneuver and look, listen, and feel for respirations. If respirations are nonexistent or agonal (less than 6/minute) then artificial respirations must be administered.
5. Begin artificial respirations. Administer two slow deep breaths while pinching the patient's nose.
6. If the airway is obstructed give six to ten back blows and sweep out the mouth with a finger until the obstruction is cleared.
7. Assess circulation by palpating the ipsilateral carotid pulse for 5 to 10 seconds.

One-Person CPR

8. If there is no pulse, begin external chest compressions in the cycle of 15 compressions and then two breaths at a rate of 80–100 per minute (15 compressions/two breaths). The hand is placed on the lower half of the sternum and compressions are 1½ to 2 inches in depth.
9. Pause after one minute to check pulse and respirations. If they are still absent, continue the cycle and pause every 5 minutes to check pulse and respiration.

Two-Person CPR

10. Begin compressions with five compressions for each breath at a rate of 80/minute.
11. Pause at 1 minute to check for pulse and respirations. If still absent, continue the cycle and pause every 5 minutes to check pulse and respiration.

Child CPR
Same as the adult, except

1. Use less force for respirations.
2. Use heel of one hand only for compressions and compress 1–1½ inches.

Infant CPR
Same as adult, except

1. Palpate brachial instead of carotid pulse.
2. Use only two fingers to compress the sterum ½–1 inch.
3. Compress at a point one finger width below the internipple line.
4. Use only puffs of air, not full breaths.

BIBLIOGRAPHY

Bates, Barbara. 1979. *A guide to physical examination.* Philadelphia: J.B. Lippincott.

Prior, J., J. Silberstein, and J. Stang. 1981. *Physical diagnosis: The history and examination of the patient.* 6th ed. St. Louis: C.V. Mosby Co.

III
Differential Diagnosis

12

Rheumatology

INTRODUCTION

Certainly, arthritis and related disorders are the most commonly encountered diseases in clinical chiropractic practice. Degenerative joint disease probably accounts for fully half of the complaints of chiropractic patients. The study of connective tissue disorders is extensive and this chapter is by no means exhaustive.

It is the purpose of this chapter to outline the more common rheumatologic disorders, including their etiology, diagnosis, and treatment, both medical and chiropractic. Disease categories as well as precise history and physical examination procedures are also outlined.

CLASSIFICATION OF RHEUMATOLOGIC DISEASES

There are myriad rheumatologic diseases, each of which can be grouped into one of many categories. Exhibit 12-1 gives the classification of the major joint diseases.

HISTORY

The key to the diagnosis of any connective tissue disorder is meticulous historical analysis. It is not an understatement to say that most diagnoses in this

Exhibit 12-1 Classification of Arthritides

Inflammatory arthritides
  Rheumatoid arthritis (RA)
  Seronegative spondyloarthropathies (SNSA)
  Ankylosing spondylitis (AS)
  Reiter's syndrome
  Arthritis associated with enteropathy
  Arthritis associated with psoriasis
  Cis-retinoic acid arthropathy
Crystal deposition arthropathy (CDA)
  Gouty arthritis
  Calcium pyrophosphate arthropathy (CPPD)
    (pseudogout)
  Hydroxyapatite deposition disease (HADD)
Infection
  Suppurative
  Nonsuppurative
Miscellaneous
  Erosive osteoarthritis (EOA)
  Juvenile chronic arthritis (JCA)
Non-inflammatory arthropathies
Degenerative joint disease (DJD)
  Primary osteoarthritis (primary OA)
  Secondary osteoarthritis (secondary OA)
  Traumatically induced DJD
Connective tissue arthropathies (CTA)
  Systemic lupus erythematosus (SLE)
  Progressive systemic sclerosis (PSS) (scleroderma)
  Polymyalgia rheumatica
Diffuse idiopathic skeletal hyperostosis (DISH)
Ossification of posterior longitudinal ligament (OPLL)
Neuropathic arthropathy
Nonarticular rheumatism
Endocrine diseases (with musculoskeletal complaints)
  Hyperthyroidism
  Hypothyroidism
  Hyperparathyroidism
  Cushing's syndrome
  Pituitary disorders
  Diabetes mellitus
Fibromyalgia syndrome

disease category can be made by proper history taking.

There are a number of questions that must be asked of all patients suspected of having a rheumatologic disease. The proper questions are illustrated below; diseases indicated by positive responses are noted parenthetically. It must be remembered that the diseases mentioned are generalizations and that there are some exceptions to these rules.

1. Sex of the patient?
   Female? (RA, primary/erosive OA, DJD)
   Male? (SNSA, DJD)
2. Is the disease monarticular? (infection, acute trauma [synovitis], chronic trauma [DJD], CDA)
3. Is the disease polyarticular? (inflammatory arthropathy, DJD, CTA)
4. Is the disease symmetric? (RA, CTA)
   Asymmetric? (DJD, SNSA, CDA, traumatic arthropathy)

Other questions that can lead to a more exact etiology of the patients complaint include:

1. Has the patient had a recent surgery (including tooth extraction) or is there a history of tuberculosis? (infection)
2. Has the patient had Crohn's disease, ulcerative colitis, or irritable bowel syndrome? (enteropathic arthritis)
3. Has the patient had urethritis, conjunctivitis, balanitis, or a sexually transmitted disease? (Reiter's syndrome)
4. Is there a history of skin disease? Psoriasis? (arthritis associated with psoriasis) Malar rash? (SLE)
5. Is there dysphagia? (DISH, PSS)
6. Is the patient diabetic? (neuropathic arthropathy, DISH)
7. Is the patient an alcoholic? (neuropathic arthropathy)
8. Is there a family history of arthritis?

PHYSICAL EXAMINATION

Physical examination of the joints and other connective tissues can also be very helpful in establishing a diagnosis. The following physical examination procedures should be performed on all rheumatology patients. Suggested diseases are noted below examination procedures.

1. Is there soft tissue swelling around the affected joint? If so, is it

concentric? (inflammatory arthritis, infection)
eccentric? (gouty arthritis, HADD, amyloidosis)

2. Are there firm bony nodules around the joint? (DJD)
3. Is there redness and heat at the affected joint(s)? (infection)
4. Is there a cutaneous fistula with drainage? (infection, RA)
5. Is the patient febrile? (infection)
6. Is there inflammatory ocular disease? (AS, Reiter's syndrome)
7. Is there inflammatory anal disease? (entero-pathic arthritis)
8. Are there scaly red lesions in the external auditory canal? (arthritis associated with psoriasis)
9. Are there subcutaneous nodules? (RA, HADD)
10. Is the disease primarily confined to the feet? (Reiter's syndrome, RA, gouty arthritis)
11. Is the disease primarily confined to the hands? (RA, primary OA, erosive OA, psoriatic arthritis)
12. Does the disease primarily involve
    large joints? (DJD)
    small joints? (RA)
    spine? (SNSA)

LABORATORY

The use of the clinical laboratory in the investigation of arthritides is almost requisite. In addition to stand-ard admission protocols of a complete blood count and urinalysis, the following investigations are helpful in the rheumatology patient.

- *Erythrocyte Sedimentation Rate (ESR)*—This test is a non-specific indicator of inflammation anywhere in the body. It can be used to monitor the progress of the disease and effectiveness of therapy.
- *Rheumatoid Factor (RF)*—This test is positive in most rheumatoid arthritis patients. High titres are frequently associated with more severe disease.
- *Anti-nuclear Antibodies (ANA)*—The presence of these antibodies is most often times seen in sys-temic lupus erythematosus; however, this is a relatively nonspecific test.

- *Anti-DNA Antibodies*—This is a relatively specific test for systemic lupus erythematosus.
- *LE Cell Prep*—This test is beneficial in the diagnosis of systemic lupus erythematosus.
- *HLA-B27*—This antigen test is most frequently positive with the seronegative spondyloarthropathies.
- *HLA-DR4*—This antigen test is not uncommonly seen in rheumatoid arthritis.
- *Serum Glucose*—Many patients with diffuse idiopathic skeletal hyperostosis will also have diabetes mellitus.

RADIOLOGY

The following radiographic findings are helpful in the diagnosis of arthropathy; their particular suggested diseases are listed paranthetically.

1. Is there periarticular osteopenia?
   Yes? (RA, SLE)
   No? (SNSA, CDA, DJD)
2. Is there bone erosion?
   Yes? (RA, SNSA, gouty arthritis [late in the disease])
   No? (DJD, CTA)
3. Is there bone production?
   Yes? (DJD, SNSA)
   No? (RA, CTA, CDA)
4. Are there calcified soft tissue masses?
   Yes? (CDA)
5. Is there joint space narrowing
   Concentric? (inflammatory arthritis)
   Eccentric? (DJD)
6. Is there osseous ankylosis of joints?
   Yes? (SNSA, RA [carpus/tarsus only], JCA)

RHEUMATOLOGIC DISEASES

The following is a summary of the more common rheumatologic diseases seen in chiropractic practice. The reader is referred to more in-depth texts for further study. Each of the disease outlines contains the following information: incidence (Incid:), etiology

(Etiol:), pathogenesis (Path:), history (Hx:), physical examination (PE:), laboratory (Lab:), radiology (Rad:), and treatment (Tx:).

Rheumatoid Arthritis

Incid:	Middle-aged females
Etiol:	Unknown
Path:	Pannus formation leading to joint destruction
Hx/PE/Lab:	Four of these for >6 weeks is diagnostic
	Morning stiffness > one hour
	Soft tissue swelling (3 or more joints)
	Swelling of wrist, MCP, PIP joints
	Bilaterally symmetric arthritis
	Subcutaneous nodules
	Positive rheumatoid factor (+ HLA-DR4)
	Radiographic evidence of RA in the hands/wrist
Rad:	Fusiform (concentric) soft tissue swelling
	Periarticular osteopenia
	Erosions of periarticular bone
	Concentric loss of joint space
	Subchondral cyst formation
	Atlantoaxial instability
	Facet joint erosions (cervical spine)
Tx:	NSAIDS, corticosteroids, gold, penicillamine, methotrexate, physical therapy

Ankylosing Spondylitis

Incid:	Young males
Etiol:	Unknown
Path:	Pannus formation with joint destruction (less aggressive than RA)
Hx:	Low back pain (sacroiliac and thoracolumbar)
	Progressive stiffness
	Inflammatory ocular disease
PE:	Decreased lumbar range of motion
	Thoracic kyphosis
	Lumbar hypolordosis
	Decreased chest expansion
	Aortic regurgitation
	Uveitis/iritis
Lab:	Positive HLA-B27
	Elevated ESR
	Negative rheumatoid factor
Rad:	Bilaterally symmetric sacroilitis/fusion
	Erosions at corners of vertebral bodies
	Sclerosis at corners of vertebral bodies

Thin vertical syndesmophyte formation
Bony fusion

Tx: NSAIDS, corticosteroids, manipulation, physical therapy

Arthritis Associated with Psoriasis

Incid: 30–50 males and females
Etiol: Unknown
Path: Similar to AS
Hx: Psoriasis (arthritis can precede psoriasis)
         Pain and stiffness (hands and thoraco-lumbar spine)
         Nail deformity (pitting)
         Inflammatory ocular disease
PE: Classic psoriatic skin lesions
         Uveitis/iritis/keratoconjunctivitis
         Decreased range of motion (hands and spine)
         Nail pitting
Lab: Positive HLA-B27
         Elevated ESR
         Negative rheumatoid factor
Rad: Asymmetrical sacroilitis/fusion
         Thick parasyndesmophytes
         Vertebral fusion
         DIP erosions (PIP/MCP also)
         Terminal phalangeal sclerosis
         Entirety of single digit involved
         Periosteal reaction along the metacarpal shafts
Tx: NSAIDS, corticosteroids, manipulation, physical therapy

Reiter's Syndrome

Incid: Young males
Etiol: Unknown, but may occur after a sexually transmitted disease (e.g., gonorrhea)
Path: Similar to AS
Hx: Classic triad (urethritis, conjunctivitis, arthritis) balanitis, keratoderma blennorrhagicum
         Low back pain
PE: Usually confined to spine and lower extremity
         Swelling of fingers/toes/heels
         Decreased range of motion
Lab: Positive HLA-B27
         Elevated ESR
         Negative rheumatoid factor
Rad: Erosions at calcaneus/MTPs
         Asymmetric sacroiliac erosions/fusion

Thick parasyndesmophytes

Spinal fusion

Periosteal reaction along the metatarsal shafts

Tx: NSAIDS, corticosteroids, manipulation, physical therapy

Arthritis Associated with Enteropathy

Other than a history of inflammatory bowel disease, enteropathic arthritis can resemble any of the SNSAs.

Gouty Arthritis

Incid: Middle-aged males

Etiol: Synovial deposition of monosodium urate crystals

Path: Crystals induce an inflammatory arthropathy

Hx: Sudden onset of excruciating monarticular arthralgia

Affects great toe most commonly (podagra)

Lumps and bumps around affected joint(s)

Fever/chills

Alcohol abuse

PE: Acutely inflamed joint with redness and swelling

Periarticular soft tissue masses

Soft tissue masses in the pinna of the ear

Lab: Strongly negatively birefringent crystals from joint aspirate under polarized light microscope

Elevated ESR

Negative rheumatoid factor/HLA-B27

+/− Hyperuricemia

Rad: Nonmarginal erosions of bone with overhanging edges

Eccentric soft tissue masses (+/− calcification)

Severe joint destruction

May be 10–12 years before any radiographic findings

Tx: Colchicine; allopurinol; NSAIDS; increased fluid intake (prevents gouty nephropathy), avoidance of alcohol, purine containing foods, caffeinated beverages, chocolate/cocoa

Calcium Pyrophosphate Crystal Deposition Disease

Incid: Adults

Etiol: Deposition of calcium pyrophosphate dihydrate crystals in joints

Path:	Crystals induce a destructive synovitis
Hx:	Usually an acute monarthritis
	Can be chronic pseudo-DJD pattern
	Occurs in joints not usually affected by DJD
	Pain/swelling/stiffness
PE:	Similar to any inflammatory arthritis
Lab:	Positively birefringent crystals from joint aspirate under polarized microscopy
	+/− Elevated ESR
	Negative rheumatoid factor
	Negative HLA-B27
Rad:	Chondrocalcinosis
	DJD in a joint that does not normally have DJD
Tx:	Joint aspiration, NSAIDS, manipulation, physical therapy

Hydroxypatite Deposition Disease

Incid:	Adult males and females
Etiol:	Hydroxyapatite crystal deposition
Path:	Crystal deposition in inflamed tendons and ligaments
Hx:	Chronic tendinitis/bursitis/enthesitis
	Old/chronic trauma
PE:	Tender ligaments and/or tendons
	+/− Palpate soft tissue mass in painful area
Lab:	+/− Elevated ESR
Rad:	Calcification in a tendon, ligament, or bursa
Tx:	NSAIDS, physical therapy (especially ultrasound)

Degenerative Joint Disease

Incid:	Older males and females
Etiol:	Chronic "wear and tear"
Path:	Dehydration, fibrillation, and degeneration of articular cartilage
Hx:	Chronic pain and stiffness
	Most common in spine and large joints of lower extremities
	May cause signs and symptoms of spinal canal stenosis
	Single joint is suggestive of traumatic induction
PE:	Decreased range of motion
	Periarticular bony nodules
	+/− Mild swelling
Lab:	Noncontributory in most cases
Rad:	Eccentric loss of joint space

Subchondral sclerosis
Subchondral cyst formation
Osteophyte formation
Erosions in hands with EOA

Tx: Manipulation, physical therapy,
        NSAIDS, surgery (arthroplasty, lami-
        nectomy, foraminotomy)

Diffuse Idiopathic Skeletal Hyperostosis

Incid: Middle-aged males
Etiol: Unknown
Path: Ossifying diathesis
Hx: Chronic spinal stiffness
        +/− Pain
PE: Decreased range of motion
        Altered spinal contours
Lab: +/− Hyperglycemia
Rad: Flowing anterolateral thick syndesmo-
        phytes that bridge vertebral bodies
        Relative preservation of disc heights
        Sparring of the facet joints
        +/− Ossification of the posterior longitu-
        dinal ligament
Tx: Manipulation
        Physical therapy
        Exercise

Fibromyalgia Syndrome

Incid: Female of childbearing age
Etiol: Unkown
Path: Fibrous infiltration of muscles
Hx: Emotional stress
        Chronic fatigue
        Diffuse stiffness/pain
        Sleep disturbance
PE: Palpation of the following points will
        elicit tenderness bilaterally:

- Nuchal line of occiput

- Mid-upper trapezius

- Scapular insertion of the rhomboids

- Pectoralis major at second costoster-
  nal area

- Bicipital groove

- Distal to lateral epicondyle at the
  elbow

- Gluteus maximus at lateral iliac crest

- One-inch posterior to greater trochanter

- L4/L5 interspinous ligament

- Pes anserine bursa
- Gastrocnemius/Achilles tendon junction

The following control points should not be tender:
  - Mid-forehead
  - Mid-ventral forearm
  - Thumbnail
  - Anterior thigh musculature

Lab: Negative rheumatoid factor
Negative ANA/LE cell prep
Negative HLA-B27
Rad: Noncontributory
Tx: Manipulation
Physical therapy
NSAIDS

BIBLIOGRAPHY

Beary, J., C. Christian, and T. Sculco, eds. 1981. *Manual of rheumatology and outpatient orthopedic disorders.* Boston: Little, Brown & Co.

Chapman, S., and R. Nakielny. 1990. *Aids to radiologic differential diagnosis.* Philadelphia: Bailliere Tindall.

Dornbrand, L., A. Hoole, R. Fletcher, and G. Pickard. 1985. *Manual of clinical problems in adult ambulatory care.* Boston: Little, Brown & Co.

Eideken, J. 1975. Arthritis. The role of the primary care physician and the radiologist. *JAMA* 232:1364.

Lawrence, J., J. Brenner, and F. Bier. 1966. Osteoarthrosis prevalence in the population and relationship between symptoms and x-ray changes. *Ann Rheum Dis* 25:1.

Pearson, C.M. 1975. Diagnosis and treatment of erosive rheumatoid arthritis and other forms of joint destruction. *Ann Intern Med* 82:241.

Simpkin, P. 1977. The pathogenesis of podagra. *Ann Intern Med* 86:230.

Yochum, T., and L. Rowe. 1987. *Essentials of skeletal radiology.* Baltimore: Williams & Wilkins Co.

13

Clinical Oncology

INTRODUCTION

The diagnosis of cancer has, in past years, been associated with terminal illness. With recent advances in chemotherapy and radiation therapy, the mortality rates with certain types of cancers have become amazingly low. One of the most beneficial aspects of cancer therapy is early diagnosis. This chapter will explain some of the most widely used methods of screening for cancer in various organ systems and also the best diagnostic methods for determining whether a patient has cancer.

SCREENING METHODS

Screening examinations must yield a significant amount of information that will benefit the patient, even if the disease is found early in its course. (Exhibit 13-1 lists cancer screening methods.) They must also be reasonably priced. After all, the primary focus is to find disease when it is clinically asymptomatic. All of the recommendations in this section are taken from a compilation of a number of references.

Table 13-1 Cancer Screening Methods

Type of Cancer	Screening Method
Central nervous system cancer	None available
Lung cancer	None available
Colon cancer	Rectal examination
	Endoscopy
	Hemoccult
Breast cancer	Self-examination
	Physician examination
	Mammogram
Prostate cancer	Rectal examination
	Ultrasound
Genital cancer (female)	Pelvic examination
	Ultrasound
	Pap smear
Genital cancer (male)	Self-examination
	Physician examination

Lung Cancer

One of the most widely used screening examinations in health care circles was the routine chest radiograph. The use of this tool as a screening method has been abandoned in recent years. There are no clinically reliable methods of screening for lung cancer.

Colon Cancer

It has been said that many colon malignancies should be palpable on digital rectal examination. For this reason, this examination should be performed in all patients over 40 years of age on a yearly basis. Testing for occult blood in the stool (stool guaiac) is recommended every year for all persons over the age of 50 and sigmoidoscopy should be performed every 3–5 years in patients over 50.

Breast Cancer

Second only to lung cancer, cancer of the breast is a leading cause of mortality in American females. Three types of examinations are useful. Self-examination of the breasts is recommended every month in all females over age 20. Examination by a doctor is recommended every three years in females age 20–40 years of age and every year thereafter. Mammography, especially with the advent of low kilovoltage techniques, is again becoming popular. A baseline study should be performed between the ages of 35 and 39 and every year in all females over 50. Frequency of mammograms between the ages of 40 and 49 should be every 1–2 years.

Genital Cancer

Uterine and ovarian cancers account for many deaths in females each year. A Pap test should be performed every 3 years in patients who have had two successive negative yearly examinations, and more often in high-risk females. This examination should begin at age 18 or when the patient becomes sexually active, whichever is earlier. Pelvic examination in females aged 20–40 should be performed every 3 years and then yearly in females over 40.

CLINICAL EXAMINATION

The clinical examination is the first line of defense in the investigation of a patient with suspected cancer. Symptoms and signs that are indicative of cancer in each organ system are outline below. Weight loss, malaise, and anorexia symptoms are found in almost all forms of cancer.

Bladder

A history of chronic cystitis along with a palpable suprapubic mass, suprapubic pain, and urethral discharge traditionally are found with bladder cancer.

Brain

Changes in personality, usually recognized by family members, and headaches are common signs of intracranial space-occupying lesions. Seizures that are focal (i.e., involve one limb or a single body region) are also an ominous sign of cerebral tumor. Visual field defects signify an intracranial mass; the type of defect also helps localize the mass. Loss of motor, bowel, and bladder control, syncope, and altered deep tendon reflexes may also signify brain tumors. The presence of pathologic reflexes is a sign of an upper motor neuron lesion as well.

Spinal Cord

Dermatomal defects, loss of motor control, altered deep tendon reflexes, and the presence of pathologic reflexes should prompt suspicion of an intracanilicular space-occupying mass.

Bone

The signs and symptoms that are most suggestive of osseous malignancy include deep unrelenting bone pain unrelieved by position or salicylates; and acute focal pain after minimal trauma, which is suggestive of pathologic fracture and diffuse skeletal pain.

Breast

A hard, immovable, nontender mass, especially located in the upper outer quadrant of the breast, with or without skin dimpling, nipple retraction and/or nipple discharge, and skin ulceration, should be regarded as malignant until proven otherwise. The presence of a family history positive for breast cancer should make the female patient regard any changes in the breast with suspicion.

Lung

The most unfortunate aspect of lung cancer is that it is usually asymptomatic until metastasis has already occurred. By that time, the prognosis for cure is poor. Signs and symptoms that are common to lung cancer include hemoptysis, cough, hoarseness, chest pain, and persistent or recurrent pneumonia.

Genital (Female)

Dysmenorrhea, dyspareunia, abnormal menstruation, a pelvic mass, vaginal discharge, a cervical mass, and a positive family history of genital cancer are strong indicators of cancer, especially in patients over the age of 40.

Genital (Male)

The presence of testicular pain, penile discharge, dysuria, difficulty starting the urinary stream, and a nontender, hard scrotal mass should prompt suspicion of malignancy.

Colon

Colon cancer is a leading cause of death in older persons in the United States. Signs and symptoms consistent with this diagnosis include abdominal pain with or without a mass, bloating, alternating diarrhea and constipation, hematochezia, and melena.

Liver

Most forms of hepatic carcinoma are invasive and, as such, do not cause signs and symptoms until late in the course of the disease. When they are present, abdominal pain, jaundice (especially when painless), and hepatomegaly are ominous signs.

Pancreas

The classic triad of abdominal pain, jaundice, and weight loss are the most common findings associated with pancreatic carcinoma. Signs of duodenal obstruction can also be present.

Kidney

An abdominal mass, flank pain, and hematuria, especially when painless, should prompt an investigation for renal carcinoma.

Stomach

Gastric cancer, although not as commonly found in the United States as in the Far East, carries with it a poor prognosis. The appearance of epigastric pain, melena, bloody vomitus, a gastric ulcer that does not heal, and dyspepsia should be regarded with suspicion for malignant change.

Leukemia

Leukemia most often affects young persons. Signs and symptoms include ecchymoses, hepatosplenomegaly, pallor, fever, and lymphadenopathy.

Lymphoma

A relatively young patient with a relapsing fever lymphadenopathy (which is often times painful with the ingestion of alcohol); hepatosplenomegaly; an abdominal mass; and/or a Virchow's node should be investigated for the possibility of lymphoma.

LABORATORY INVESTIGATION

Although laboratory investigation of patients with suspected cancer is often nonspecific, it can be useful and can lead the physician to other more sensitive and specific diagnostic tests. The following is a list of some diagnostic tests that are helpful. Specific reference values should be sought from your particular laboratory.

- *Hemoccult*—Tests the patient's stool for the presence of blood; three consecutive positive tests are necessary for definitive diagnosis; helpful in the diagnosis of gastrointestinal malignancy
- *Carcinoembryonic Antigen*—Nonspecific but useful in the diagnosis of carcinoma of the colon, pancreas, lung, and stomach; also increased in smokers and with hepatic and inflammatory bowel diseases

- *Alpha-fetoprotein*—Nonspecific but useful in the diagnosis of hepatic carcinoma and testicular carcinoma
- *Human Chorionic Gonadotropin*—Useful in the diagnosis of testicular tumors and choriocarcinoma; also elevated with pregnancy
- *Prostate Specific Antigen*—Useful in the diagnosis of prostate cancer but also elevated with benign prostatic hypertrophy in some cases
- *Alkaline Phosphatase*—Elevated with bone malignancy, especially blastic forms
- *Acid Phosphatase*—Elevated with prostate malignancy but also with other prostate diseases and medullary replacement disorders
- *Protein Electrophoresis*—Elevated albumin and gamma globulins are suggestive of multiple myeloma
- *White Blood Cell Count*—Nonspecific but severe elevation is suggestive of leukemia; Auer rods are seen with acute myelogenous leukemia
- *Calcium*—Increased with metastatic bone tumors but highly nonspecific
- *Complete Blood Count*—Nonspecific but can be an indicator of anemia and demonstrate specific cell types seen with certain malignancies

Table 13-2 lists laboratory studies that can be performed when certain types of malignancies are suspected.

Table 13-2 Laboratory Tests for Specific Malignancies

Type of Malignancy	Suggested Test
Skeletal	Calcium
	Alkaline phosphatase
	Acid phosphatase
	Protein electrophoresis
Prostate	Acid phosphatase
	Prostate specific antigen
Kidney	Urinalysis
	Complete blood count
Reticuloendothelial	Complete blood count
Colon	Hemoccult
	Complete blood count
	CEA

DIAGNOSTIC IMAGING

Although the plain film radiograph is the pillar of general clinical practice, it is usually of little help in the diagnosis of malignancy, especially in the early stages. Advanced imaging procedures such as radionuclide bone scanning, CT, and MRI are much more sensitive and specific methods in the investigation of cancer. The following list gives the most effective procedures for certain types of malignancies.

- *Skeletal Malignancy*—See Figure 13-1.
- *Lung Cancer*—See Figure 13-2. Plain film radiographs are not often diagnostic in early bronchogenic carcinoma.

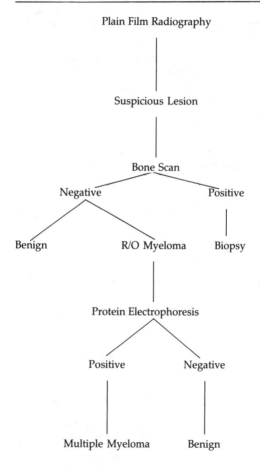

Figure 13-1 Investigation of Skeletal Malignancy

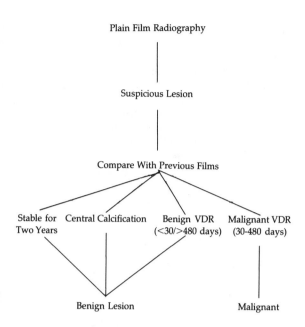

Note: If the lesion is indeterminate but probably benign, re-x-ray at 1-, 3-, 6-, 9-, 12-, and 24-month intervals for changes suggestive of malignancy. (VDR = volume doubling rate)

Figure 13-2 Investigation of Lung Cancer

- *Central Nervous System Malignancy*—MRI, with or without gadolinium contrast enhancement.
- *Hepatic, Pancreatic, Bladder, Colon, and Stomach Cancers*—CT, with or without MRI. Ultrasound and angiography can also be of some benefit in many cases.
- *Lymphomas*—Contrast enhanced CT, MRI.
- *Leukemias*—Usually require a combination of techniques, including plain film radiography, radionuclide bone scanning, CT, and MRI.

The chapter on differential diagnosis elaborates more specifically on the investigation of specific signs and symptoms that are mentioned in this chapter.

BIBLIOGRAPHY

Chapman, S., and R. Nakielny. 1990. *Aids to radiologic differential diagnosis*. Philadelphia: Bailliere Tindall.

Dornbrand, L., A. Hoole, R. Fletcher, and G. Pickard. 1985. *Manual of clinical problems in adult ambulatory care*. Boston: Little, Brown & Co.

Goroll, A., L. May, and A. Mulley. 1987. *Primary care medicine: Office evaluation and management of the adult patient*. Philadelphia: J.B. Lippincott.

McMillan, J., E. Levine, and R. Stephens. 1982. Computed tomography in the evaluation of metastatic adenocarcinoma from an unknown primary site. *Radiology* 143:143.

McNeil, B., and H. Abrams. 1986. *Brigham and Women's Hospital handbook of diagnostic imaging*. Boston: Little, Brown & Co.

14

Spine Pain

INTRODUCTION

One of the most important tasks for the chiropractic physician is to accurately diagnose the cause of the patient's neck or back pain. The list of diseases that can cause pain of this type is almost endless. This chapter describes the most common causes of spine pain, both within and outside the spinal column.

VERTEBROGENIC SPINE PAIN

The following is a list of intrinsic spine disorders that can result in pain in the spine or paraspinal regions. (Exhibit 14-1 lists vertobrogenic causes of spine pain.)

Arthritides

- *Ankylosing Spondylitis (AS)*—This disease begins by causing pain in the sacroiliac joints, usually bilaterally, and then progresses to the thoracolumbar spine, and cephalically and caudally from that point forward.
- *Degenerative Disc Disease (DDD)*—Chronic, dull, achy pain is the hallmark of DDD. Pain can be radiating in cases when spinal canal stenosis has developed, but can improve with a flexed posture, such as when riding a bicycle.

Exhibit 14-1 Common Vertebrogenic Causes of Spine Pain

Arthritides	Infectious
AS	Brucellosis
DDD	Coccidioidomycosis
DISH	E. coli
Aseptic diskitis	Pseudomonas
Enteropathic arthritis	Tuberculosis
Facet arthrosis	Metabolic
Psoriatic arthritis	Hyperparathyroidism
Reiter's syndrome	Osteoporosis
RA	Miscellaneous
Chiropractic	Fibrous dysplasia
Hypermobility	Paget's disease
Hypomobility	Trauma
Myofascitis	Disc bulge/HNP
Subluxation	Fracture/dislocation
Developmental	Facet syndrome
Basilar invagination	Spondylolisthesis
Block vertebrae	Sprain/strain
Dysplasias	Tumors
Transitional segments	Benign
Miscellaneous	Malignant

- *Diffuse Idiopathic Skeletal Hyperostosis (DISH)*—The pain of this disease is mild and nonspecific in most cases. If ossification of the posterior longitudinal ligament is also present, signs of spinal canal stenosis can prevail.

- *Diskitis (aseptic)*—Often found in young persons, this disease most often presents with moderate to severe focal thoracic spine pain. A calcified disc may be noted radiographically.

- *Enteropathic Arthritis*—The pain of this disease is similar to AS, although lower extremity complaints along with spine pain are more common.

- *Osteoarthritis of the Facet Articulations*—Local pain at the level(s) of degeneration along with radiating pain, usually not beyond the elbow or knee, are the common presentations.

- *Psoriatic Arthritis*—Again, pain is similar to AS, but concomitant hand pain is also seen.

- *Reiter's Syndrome*—Pain in the heels and feet usually accompany low back and sacroiliac pain.

- *Rheumatoid Arthritis (RA)*—Most often this disease involves chronic pain, with periodic acute exacerbations, in the cervical spine.

Chiropractic

- *Intervertebral Hypermobility*—Pain can be localized to a single level or may radiate, but not usually below mid-extremity.
- *Intervertebral Hypomobility*—pain is similar to hypermobility except that stiffness accompanies the pain.
- *Myofascitis*—Muscle pain adjacent to the spine is common with many of the diseases in this category.
- *Subluxation*—This lesion can cause focal or diffuse spine pain, radiating pain not below the elbow or knee, and/or referred pain to visceral structures.

Developmental

- *Basilar Invagination*—The pain of this condition is usually suboccipital in nature, but there may be referral of the pain into the extremities and down the spine as well.
- *Block Vertebrae*—The hypermobility above and below a synostotic segment causes pain, as other forms of hypermobility will.
- *Congenital Dysplasias*—(e.g., Marfan's syndrome). The pain seen with these diseases is dependent upon the disease present and its severity.
- *Lumbosacral Transitional Segments*—Focal lumbosacral pain, with or without radiation, is the traditional pain pattern. The pain from this anomaly can be very confusing, however.
- *Miscellaneous Vertebral Anomalies*—(e.g., hemivertebra). Pain patterns are dependent upon the anomaly present.
- *Occipitocervical Transitional Segments*—Just as with lumbosacral transitional segments, the pain pattern can be very confusing. It can cause focal spine pain, radiating pain, and even headaches.

Infectious

- *Brucellosis*—After exposure, usually to cattle feces, the slow onset of pain and stiffness become apparent. This disease rarely affects the spine.
- *Coccidioidomycosis*—The pain of this fungus is usually localized to an apophysis. The lungs are the primary route of infections and the spine becomes involved when there is dissemination.
- *E. coli*—This infection can result from septicemia from another infection or in drug abusers.
- *Pseudomonas*—This is another infection seen in intravenous drug abusers. Pain is insidious in onset and chronic in nature.
- *Tuberculosis*—Tuberculosis of the spine can be very devastating, with severe destruction of the discs and vertebrae and a resultant gibbus deformity.

Metabolic

- *Hyperparathyroidism*—The pain from this condition is usually located in the sacroiliac joints, although when there is bone resorption in the vertebral bodies pain is felt there as well.
- *Osteoporosis*—Osteoporosis becomes especially painful when compression fractures occur, although infractions (microfactures) of the endplates are painful as well.

Miscellaneous

- *Fibrous Dysplasia*—This lesion is usually painless unless there has been a pathologic fracture. Polyostotic forms of the disease can be painful by themselves.
- *Paget's Disease*—The pain of Paget's disease is usually chronic and may become acute if there is a pathologic fracture.

Trauma

- *Disc Bulge*—Focal pain, many times with radiation to the extremities, is the hallmark presentation.
- *Dislocation*—Acute focal pain, with myelopathy if there is instability, is the rule.
- *Facet Syndrome (synovitis)*—Focal pain at the level of involvement with radiation to the knee or elbow is common. There may also be visceral referral.
- *Fracture*—Pain is very similar to a dislocation.
- *Herniated Nucleus Pulposus*—Focal back or neck pain with dermatomal radiation to the hands or feet is the most common presentation. The cauda equine syndrome can be the result of a large central disc herniation.
- *Spondylolisthesis*—The pain of this lesion is often times an enigma. No specific pain pattern is extremely common, but bilateral buttock pain is not uncommon.
- *Sprain/Strain*—Focal muscular and vertebral pain is most common, although there can be some mild radiation of the pain.

Tumors

- *Benign Tumors*—The pain of benign spinal tumors is usually focal and unless the tumor is expansible and causes spinal canal stenosis, there is little or no radiation of pain. Types of benign tumors include aneurysmal bone cyst, giant cell tumor (quasimalignant), osteoblastoma, and osteoid osteoma, and hemangioma (most common/rarely painful).
- *Malignant Tumors*
  Chordoma—The pain from this tumor is usually localized to the sacrum, as this is the most common location in the spine.
  Metastasis—The pain of this condition can be focal or diffuse depending upon the extent of the disease. In either event, the pain is chronic and unrelieved by changes in position.
  Multiple Myeloma—The pain of this reticuloendothelial malignancy is very similar to the pain of metastasis.

REFERRED SPINE PAIN

There are a number of nonspinal disorders that may refer pain to the spine and paraspinal structures. This clinical presentation can be quite confusing. When the clinician is directed to a pattern of referred pain from the history and physical examination, the following list of differential diagnoses, grouped by the region to which each of them refers pain, will be helpful. (These are summarized in Table 14-1).

Cervical Spine

- *Brain Lesions*—All of these lesions cause diffuse pain referred to the cervical spine. Spinal stiffness

Table 14-1 Diseases That Commonly Refer Pain to the Spine

Spinal Location	Disease
Cervical	Brain lesions
	CAD
	Dental disease
	Esophageal disease
	Upper airway disease
	Lymphadenopathy
Thoracic	Aortic aneurysm
	CAD
	CHF
	Gallbladder disease
	Herpes zoster
	Hiatal hernia
	Kidney disease
	Lung disease
	Pancreatic disease
	Peptic ulcer disease
	Rib lesions
	Spinal cord tumor
Lumbar	Aortic aneurysm
	Colon cancer
	Endometriosis
	Hip disease
	Kidney disease
	Ovarian disease
	PID
	Pregnancy
	Short leg syndrome
	Spinal cord tumor
	Uterine cancer

may accompany infection and hemorrhage, as well. Causes of brain lesions include arteriovenous malformations, aneurysm, cerebrovascular accident, infection, subarachnoid hemorrhage, subdural hematoma, and tumors.

- *Coronary Artery Disease* (CAD)—The pain of myocardial ischemia is usually referred to the left neck and jaw.
- *Dental Caries/Periodontal Abscess*—Pain is usually referred to the upper cervical spine.
- *Esophageal Disease*—The location of pain is dependent upon the location of the esophageal lesion.
- *Laryngeal/Pharyngeal Disease*—Pain can be referred to anywhere in the cervical region.
- *Lymphadenopathy*—Focal pain is usually noted in the area of the enlarged lymph nodes.
- *Pancoast Tumor*—Cervicothoracic pain is usually the rule.
- *Temporomandibular Joint Disease*—Just as with many other disorders, the pain referral pattern is nonspecific.

Thoracic Spine

- *Aortic Aneurysm*—Mid-back pain, severe with a dissecting type, is most often seen.
- *Coronary Artery Disease*—Pain referred to the mid-back is not uncommon.
- *Congestive Heart Failure* (CHF)—This can, but does not often, refer pain to the thoracic region.
- *Gall Bladder Disease*—Pain is usually referred to the right paraspinal region near the tip of the scapula.
- *Herpes Zoster*—A dermatomal referral pattern associated with the level involved is the traditional pattern.
- *Hiatal Hernia*—Dull achy pain can be referred to the mid-back.
- *Kidney Disease*—Pain is usually felt in the costovertebral angle(s).
- *Lung Diseases*—Any lung disease can refer pain to the thoracic region. Such diseases can include malignancy, pneumonia, and mediastinal masses.

- *Pancreatic Disease*—These lesions usually refer straight through to the lower thoracic region. The pain can be very severe. Such diseases can include malignancy, pancreatitis, and pseudocyst.
- *Peptic Ulcer Disease*—This condition can cause sharp pain in the lower thoracic region.
- *Rib Lesions*—Lesions of the posterior ribs, such as from fractures or tumors, can result in local and radiating spine pain.
- *Spinal Cord Tumor*—Focal pain at the affected level and radiating pain above and, more commonly, below the lesion are common.

Lumbar Spine

- *Aortic Aneurysm*—Focal or diffuse pain in the region of the dilatation are not uncommon.
- *Colorectal Cancer*—Referred pain to the paraspinal regions is not unheard of.
- *Endometriosis*—The referred pain of endometriosis is dependent upon the location of the lesions.
- *Hip Disease*—These lesions can refer pain to the low back.
- *Kidney Disease*—Pain is usually noted at the costovertebral angle(s). Causes can include infection, stones, and tumors.
- *Ovarian Disease*—These conditions can refer dull, achy pain to the low back and pelvis.
- *Pelvic Inflammatory Disease (PID)*—Just as with endometriosis, the referral pattern is dependent upon the location of the disease.
- *Pregnancy*—Low back and sacroiliac pain from ligamentous laxity are relatively common sequelae of pregnancy.
- *Short Leg Syndrome*—Pain patterns are nonspecific but are usually due to altered biomechanics in the low back.
- *Spinal Cord Tumors*—Focal pain, with or without radiation, is not uncommon. The tumors can be gliomas, meningiomas, or metastatis.
- *Uterine Cancer*—Dull, achy low back and pelvic pain is not uncommon.

BIBLIOGRAPHY

Beary, J., C. Christian, and T. Sculco, eds. 1981. *Manual of rheumatology and outpatient orthopedic disorders*. Boston: Little, Brown & Co.

Chapman, S., and R. Nakielny. 1990. *Aids to radiologic differential diagnosis*. Philadelphia: Bailliere Tindall.

Hager, H. 1990. *Normal biomechanical stresses in spinal function*. Gaithersburg, Md.: Aspen Publishers, Inc.

Ruge, D. 1977. *Spinal disorders: Diagnosis and treatment*. Philadelphia: Lea and Febiger.

15

Differential Diagnosis

INTRODUCTION

Differential diagnosis is an art that should be perfected by all practitioners of the healing arts. It involves the development of a list of causes for a collated group of findings. The list is then organized from most likely to least likely and then shortened by the exclusion (rule out [R/O]) of certain diagnoses through the use of diagnostic tests. In this way, the most probable final diagnosis is reached and appropriate treatment is instituted.

This chapter will specify some of the most common causes for many of the symptoms, signs, and findings in chiropractic clinical practice.

Remember, if you hear hoofbeats, think of horses and not zebras.

It is useful to recall that the most common diseases happen most commonly; think of them first. An asterisk in the text identifies something that may not be the most common cause for a finding but something that should be the first thing ruled out in the list of differential diagnoses, as it is usually the most ominous, if not life-threatening.

The best techniques for the investigation of the noted abnormalities are enumerated after the list of differential diagnoses.

ABDOMEN

Adrenal Calcification

Calcification of the adrenal gland usually occurs secondarily to some form of inflammatory disease.

Trauma, usually birth trauma, is by far the most common cause for adrenal calcification, followed by cancer* and infection of the adrenal gland. The investigation of adrenal calcification is best accomplished with CT.

Dysphagia

Dysphagia is the inability to swallow objects without difficulty. It usually begins with difficulty with liquids and progresses to solids. It has both organic and psychological causes.

Cancer,* whether intrinsic esophageal or extrinsic from some other regional organ, is a common cause of dysphagia. Primary achalasia, reflux esophagitis with stricture, and hypertrophic spinal diseases (such as diffuse idiopathic skeletal hyperostosis and degenerative disc disease) are also common etiologies for dysphagia. Globus hystericus is a condition where there is no true esophageal luminal stricture but a sensation of dysphagia. It is a diagnosis made after the exclusion of other causes.

Contrast examination with barium sulfate of the upper gastrointestinal tract and endoscopy are helpful techniques in the study of this complaint. Plain film radiography will help outline hypertrophic spinal diseases.

Hematemesis

Vomiting of blood can be a sign of ominous disease such as cancer,* but it also may be a sign of simple peptic ulcer disease or gastritis. Esophageal varices are a common cause of hematemesis in alcoholic patients.

Analysis of hematemesis with endoscopy and upper gastrointestinal barium sulfate contrast examination will usually yield sufficient information to make a diagnosis.

Hematochezia

The passage of bright red blood per rectum is most often caused by hemorrhoids, although inflammatory bowel disease (such as ulcerative colitis, irritable bowel syndrome, and Crohn's disease), cancer of the rectum,* and intestinal polyps are relatively common etiologies as well.

Barium enema, upper gastrointestinal series, and endoscopy are the most commonly utilized procedures in the investigation of bloody stool.

Hepatomegaly

Cirrhosis, whether alcoholic or otherwise, hepatitis, cancer,* and congestive heart failure can all cause enlargement of the liver. Many times biopsy is the only definitive procedure which will identify the cause of the enlargement.

The investigation of hepatomegaly should begin with an ultrasound examination of the abdomen, possibly followed by more invasive procedures, such as endoscopic retrograde cholangiopancreatography or percutaneous transhepatic cholangiography. Both procedures risk infection and should be reserved for patients with the appropriate clinical indications. CT and CT-guided biopsy of the liver can also be helpful.

Abdominal Mass (Adult)

Saccular abdominal aortic aneurysms, pregnancy, ovarian cysts and tumors, renal masses, and gallbladder disease are the most common causes of abdominal masses in adults. The absence of any abnormality is also a common finding when the initial abdominal mass is investigated. The presence of colon cancer* should always be excluded in the appropriate age group as well.

The primary, albeit cursory, examination for an abdominal mass is the plain film radiographic investigation. This is usually followed by US and CT.

Melena

Black tarry stools are a sign that there is gastrointestinal bleeding proximal to the mid-transverse colon. A patient over the age of 40, with melena, usually in conjunction with anemia, is often significant for colon cancer. Inflammatory bowel diseases, including peptic ulcer disease and intestinal polyps, are relatively common causes as well.

The investigation of melena is very similar to the investigation of hematochezia.

Pancreatic Calcification

Chronic pancreatitis, usually secondary to alcoholism, is the most common etiology for calcification of the pancreas. Pancreatic pseudocyst and cancer of the pancreas* are also causes.

The investigation of pancreatic calcification is undertaken with CT and US procedures. Endoscopic retrograde cholangiopancreatography may also be helpful in certain instances.

Pneumoperitoneum

Air in the peritoneal cavity most often occurs after abdominal surgery. Perforation of a hollow viscus, such as occurs with a perforated peptic ulcer or other inflammatory bowel disease (such as diverticulitis), is also a common cause. Introduction of air per vagina, as occurs with douching, can also result in a pneumoperitoneum. There is also an idiopathic form.

The investigation of air in the peritoneal cavity begins with plain film radiographic examination in the upright and lateral decubitus postures, if the positions are comfortable for the patient. If perforation is suspected, contrast examination may be indicated.

Renal Calcification

By far, the most common cause of renal calcification is the presence of a renal calculus (stone). Infection and cancer* are less common causes, as are intrinsic inflammatory diseases of the kidney, such as renal papillary necrosis.

US and CT are the most helpful techniques in the investigation of renal calcification.

Splenic Calcification

Splenic artery atherosclerosis and/or aneurysm, splenic cysts, healed hematoma, and infarction, especially in sickle cell anemia patients, are some of the more common reasons for calcification in the spleen.

Splenomegaly

Leukemias and lymphomas,* infections, and portal hypertension are common causes of an enlarged spleen. Splenomegaly often accompanies hepatomegaly. Diseases causing an enlarged liver should also be included in the list of differential diagnoses.

The investigation of splenic diseases, including calcifications, usually begins with plain film radiography and may also include US and CT.

Vas Deferens Calcification

Diabetes mellitus is the most common cause of vas deferens calcification. There is also an idiopathic form in which infection may be an etiology.

Investigation is usually performed with US, although more invasive contrast techniques are available.

CHEST

Consolidation

Consolidation of the pulmonary parenchyma is defined as the filling of the alveoli with a substance, usually blood, pus, water, or cells. Collapse of the alveoli, atelectasis, may cause a similar configuration. This pattern is also known as a pulmonary infiltrate. Causes include pulmonary edema, typically from congestive heart failure, and pneumonia. Malignant causes include lymphoma and alveolar cell carcinoma.* The two diseases will fail to respond to antibiotic or diuretic therapy as the others would.

Investigation of consolidation is classically performed with plain film radiography. Biopsy or bronchial lavage may be necessary in cases of suspected malignancy.

Effusion

Fluid in the pleural space is most frequently seen with congestive heart failure. Infection and cancer,* especially lymphangitic metastasis, are also common etiologies.

Plain film radiography is again the mainstay in investigation of this complaint, but thoracocentesis may be utilized to better define the nature of the fluid.

Extrapleural Sign

Rib metastasis, rib fracture, a loculated pleural effusion, and mesothelioma associated with asbestosis are the most frequent causes for a pleural-based, tapered bordered lesion. It must be recognized that these lesions are not within the lung parenchyma.

Plain film radiography and CT are essential in the investigation of these diseases.

Hilar Enlargement (Bilateral)

Enlargement of the lymph nodes of the hila is regularly caused by diseases such as lymphoma (especially Hodgkin's disease), sarcoidosis, lymphangitic metastasis, and infections such as tuberculosis.

Evaluation of bilateral hilar enlargement, after plain film radiography, is usually accomplished with contrast-enhanced CT scans.

Hilar Enlargement (Unilateral)

The diseases associated with unilateral enlargement of a hilum are similar to those seen with bilateral enlargement except that bronchogenic carcinoma and vascular diseases are also included.

Investigation of these diseases is the same as with bilateral hilar enlargement except that angiography is added when the lesion is assumed to be vascular.

Mediastinal Mass (Anterior)

The five "Ts" of anterior mediastinal masses are the thymoma, teratoma, thyroid (substernal), terrible aortic aneurysm, and terrible lymphoma. It is worthwhile understanding that the etiology of any mediastinal mass is secondary to the location of the mass. For example, as there are many lymph nodes in the anterior mediastinum and few in the posterior mediastinum, lymphomas occur most commonly in the anterior compartment.

Classification of the abnormality depends on the suspected etiology but CT is the mainstay advanced imaging procedure. It should be performed with contrast.

Mediastinal Mass (Middle)

Lymphoma, bronchogenic carcinoma, bronchogenic cyst, and aortic aneurysm are the four most frequent causes of a middle mediastinal mass.

Again, CT is the primary advanced imaging procedure. Angiography may be utilized if an aortic aneurysm is suspected.

Mediastinal Mass (Posterior)

Since the posterior mediastinum is in close approximation to the spine, neurogenic tumors are the most common cause of masses in this region. Aortic aneurysm, hiatal hernia, and neurenteric cyst with or without vertebral anomalies are also demonstrated.

Investigation with CT is helpful.

Multiple Pulmonary Nodules

Metastasis is the most common cause of multiple pulmonary nodules in the older patient. Old infections, especially tuberculosis and fungal disease, are common causes in the younger age group. They are also very traditionally calcified.

Plain film radiography is the primary investigational technique while CT, with or without biopsy, is often used.

Unresolving Pneumonia

Pneumonia that is slow to resolve or fails to resolve with therapy should be considered of a malignant etiology until proven otherwise. Other causes include improper therapy and benign bronchial obstruction.

Tomography, whether plain film or computerized, is helpful in finding an obstructing lesion in the lung.

Solitary Pulmonary Nodule

Bronchogenic carcinoma, infectious or noninfectious granuloma, metastasis, and benign tumors are traditionally the most common causes of a solitary small round pulmonary parenchymal lesion.

Evaluation begins with a comparison of the most recent chest radiographs with any taken in the past. If there has been an increase in the size of the lesion, especially if the volume of the lesion has doubled within 1 to 18 months, then malignancy is the prime concern. If the lesion has remained stable for two years or more, it can be considered benign. Advanced imaging with CT is helpful in finding calcifications within the lesion, which most often signify a benign etiology.

NERVOUS SYSTEM

Anisocoria

Pupillary inequality can be an enigma. Normal variants of the eye, Horner's syndrome, cranial nerve III palsy, a damaged iris, drug ingestion, brain tumor,* and cerebral ischemia are just a few of the common causes.

Investigation begins with physical examination and may also include cerebral MRI or CT with contrast to rule out a brain tumor or cerebral ischemia; laboratory investigation for ingested drugs; or a chest film to rule out a Pancoast's tumor in the lung apex.

Bitemporal Hemianopia

Pituitary tumors, optic chiasm tumors (such as meningiomas), hypothalamic masses, and a chordoma of the clivus are some of the more common causes for this finding.

Advanced imaging with CT if a bone lesion is suspected or MRI if a soft tissue lesion is suspected are helpful modalities.

Dementia

Alzheimer's disease (presenile dementia, Alzheimer's type), other forms of senility, brain tumors,* hepatic disease, and vitamin deficiency are familiar etiologies.

Investigation is typically done by MRI although specialized forms of CT are also available.

Dizziness

Dizziness is a very nonspecific finding indicative of a list of diseases too detailed for this manuscript. Suffice it to say that orthostatic hypotension, cardiac arrhythmias,* anemia, cerebellar disease, drug ingestion, endocrine diseases (such as Addison's disease), carotid sinus hypersensitivity, and inner ear disease are a few of the more traditional causes.

Evaluation of dizziness is directed at the more specific cause gleaned from the history and physical examination.

Headache

Muscle tension is by far the most common cause of headaches. Increased intracranial pressure, vascular spasm and dilatation (migraine), cluster headaches, ocular disease, dental disease, trauma, ischemic vascular disease,* hemorrhage,* and tumors* have also been implicated.

Study of the cause for a patient's headache is again directed at evaluating possible causes elicited from the history and physical examination. (See Table 15-1.)

Hyperreflexia

Brain and spinal cord tumors,* trauma with hemorrhage, and demyelinating diseases (such as multiple

Table 15-1 Evaluation of Headache

Cause	Evaluating Procedure
Muscle tension	Orthopedic testing
	History
Increased intracranial pressure	Magnetic resonance imaging
	Fundoscopic examination
Ocular disease	Eye examination
	Magnetic resonance imaging
Migraine	History
Cerebral ischemia	Magnetic resonance imaging
	Angiography
Cerebral hemorrhage	Magnetic resonance imaging

sclerosis and cerebral ischemia) are the most common causes of increased deep tendon reflexes.

Evaluation of hyperreflexia is most often undertaken with MRI although CT will be helpful in cases of suspected bone disease.

Hyporeflexia

Neuropathies, whether diabetic or otherwise, radiculopathy from foraminal encroachment by osteophytes, trauma with or without syringomyelia, spinal cord tumors,* and tabes dorsalis can all result in diminished deep tendon reflexes.

If an osseous cause is suspected, CT is helpful; soft tissue lesions are best investigated with MRI.

Ophthalmoplegia

Loss of the cardinal ranges of motion of the eye can result from a myriad of causes. Cranial nerve palsies, orbital diseases (such as infection and masses), myesthenia gravis, multiple sclerosis, brain tumors,* and cerebral ischemia are a few of the more common causes.

Cranial and orbital imaging with CT and/or MRI are beneficial in the investigation of this disorder.

Peripheral Nerve Entrapment Sites

The most common peripheral nerve entrapment sites are noted in Exhibit 15-1.

Polyneuropathy

Diabetes mellitus is probably the most common cause of peripheral polyneuropathy. Other causes include multiple sclerosis, hepatic cirrhosis, Charcot-Marie-Tooth disease, infectious mononucleosis, ingestion of toxins (such as lead, arsenic, and drugs), and the Guillain-Barré syndrome.

Evaluation of a polyneuropathy is best achieved with neurodiagnostic evaluation, including electromyography, somatosensory evoked potentials, nerve conduction velocities, and advance imaging studies such as CT and MRI.

Syncope

Orthostatic hypotension, a vasovagal response of the physiologic type; autonomic neuropathies (such as diabetes mellitus); and cardiac diseases (such as arrhythmias, ischemic vascular disease, hyperventilation, and hypoglycemia) are just a few of the more common etiologies for fainting.

Again, evaluation is based upon the initial findings of the history and physical examination (see Table 15-2).

Exhibit 15-1 Peripheral Nerve Entrapment Sites

Brachial plexus at thoracic outlet
Lateral femoral cutaneous nerve at inguinal ligament
Median nerve at carpal tunnel
Peroneal nerve at fibular head
Suprascapular nerve at scapular groove
Tibial nerve at medial malleolus
Ulnar nerve at elbow
Ulnar nerve at tunnel of Guyon

Table 15-2 Evaluation of Syncope

Cause	Evaluating Procedure
Orthostatic hypotension	Blood pressures, standing and supine
	History
Diabetes/hypoglycemia	Serum glucose
Cardiac arrhythmias	Electrocardiogram
Cerebral ischemia	Magnetic resonance imaging
	Angiography

Tremors

The two most common causes for tremors are inherited physiologic tremors and Parkinsonism.

These lesions are best investigated with neurodiagnostic modalities (as outlined above) and cerebral MRI.

Vertigo

Vestibulopathy (inner ear disease), alcohol and drug intoxication, Meniere's disease, and benign paroxysmal positional vertigo should be the primary choices when investigating this complaint.

The caloric test, laboratory investigation for intoxication, and cerebral advanced imaging are the most helpful modalities when evaluating this complaint.

Weakness (Muscular)

The complaint of muscular weakness can be relatively nonspecific. Conditions that present with this disorder include myesthenia gravis, multiple sclerosis, drug ingestion, dystonias, brain tumors,* spinal cord lesions,* and peripheral nerve lesions.

Laboratory investigation for drug ingestion, MRI, and neurodiagnostic evaluation are traditionally used for evaluation of weakness.

SKELETON

Arthritis (Monarticular)

Infection* is always the primary R/O in a patient with a monarticular arthritis. Other causes include traumatic synovitis, gouty arthritis, pseudogout, and degenerative joint disease, if the arthritis is chronic.

Plain film radiography is the first procedure to be performed, but radionuclide bone scanning and indium-111 labeled leukocyte scanning can be effectively used for infection. Joint aspiration is the only procedure available to definitively arrive at a diagnosis.

Arthritis (Polyarticular)

Rheumatoid arthritis is the most common cause of inflammatory joint disease, while degenerative joint disease is the most common cause of arthritis in general. Arthritis associated with psoriasis, Reiter's syndrome, and arthritis associated with enteropathy are other common causes.

Diagnosis of polyarthritides is usually established with plain film radiography and laboratory investigation. (Chapter 12 on rheumatology is more specific in terms of diagnostic modalities.)

Pain (Diffuse)

Metastasis is the most common cause of diffuse skeletal pain, followed closely by multiple myeloma and osteoporosis.

Radionuclide bone scanning and serum calcium, alkaline phosphatase, and protein electrophoresis are good supplements to plain film radiography.

Pain (Focal Appendicular)

Fractures, dislocations, and hematomas are the most common etiologies for focal appendicular skeletal pain. Other causes include benign bone tumors (such as osteoid osteoma), giant cell tumor, and malignant skeletal tumors (such as metastasis and multiple myeloma).

Plain film radiography supplemented with CT and radionuclide bone scanning are standard for evaluating these disorders.

Pain (Focal Spine)

Subluxation, trauma, arthritis, benign bone tumors (such as giant cell tumor and osteoid osteoma), and malignant skeletal tumors* are common causes of spine pain. (Chapter 14 further elaborates on the causes for this common malady.)

Scoliosis

The most common form of scoliosis is the idiopathic form. Etiologies such as trauma, skeletal dysplasias (like Marfan's syndrome), and neuroectodermal diseases (such as neurofibromatosis) are less common causes.

Plain film radiography and genetic testing are helpful adjuncts in the evaluation of lateral curvatures of the spine.

BIBLIOGRAPHY

Branch, W. 1986. Approach to syncope. *J Gen Intern Med* 1:49.

Chapman, S., and R. Nakielny. 1990. *Aids to radiologic differential diagnosis*. Philadelphia: Bailliere Tindall.

Cope, A. 1972. *Early diagnosis of the acute abdomen*. 14th ed. London: Oxford University Press.

Drachman, D. 1972. An approach to the dizzy patient. *Neurology* 22:323.

Edwards, D. 1975. Discriminative information in the diagnosis of dysphagia. *J Royal Coll Physicians* 9:257.

Friedman, A. 1979. Nature of headache. *Headache*. 19:163.

Gomella, L., ed. 1989. *Clinician's pocket reference*. Norwalk, Conn.: Appleton & Lange.

Kelley, W., E. Harris, and S. Ruddy, eds. 1981. *Textbook of rheumatology*. Philadelphia: W.B. Saunders Co.

Mawdsley, C. 1975. Diseases of the central nervous system: Involuntary movements. *Br Med J* 4:572.

Steer, M. 1983. Diagnostic procedures in gastrointestinal hemorrhage. *N Engl J Med* 309:646.

16

Commonly Prescribed Medications with Neuromusculo-skeletal Side Effects

A number of medications can have neuromusculo-skeletal complaints as side effects. Complaints of headache (Exhibit 16-1), dizziness/vertigo (Exhibit 16-2), weakness (Exhibit 16-3), myalgia (Exhibit 16-4), and osteoporosis/fractures (Exhibit 16-5) are not uncommon with many medications. This chapter delineates some of the more commonly prescribed drugs, and their side effects, that may alter the workup of a patient presenting to the chiropractic clinician.

It is not the purpose of this chapter to list the frequency of side effects. It is instead designed to lead the reader to the diagnosis that a patient's complaint is not a true neuromusculoskeletal disease but a side effect of a drug. It must be remembered that the diagnosis of a

Exhibit 16-1 Drugs That Cause Headaches

Antidepressants
Nitrates
NSAIDS
Sedatives
Sulfonamide antibiotics
Vasodialators

Exhibit 16-2 Drugs That Cause Dizziness or Vertigo

Aminoglycoside antibiotics
Amphetamines
Antidepressants
Antivirals
NSAIDS
Polypeptide antibiotics
Tetracyclines

Exhibit 16-3 Drugs That Cause Weakness

Antihistamines
Beta blockers
Cancer chemotherapy
Diuretics
Polypeptide antibiotics
Sedatives
Sympatholytics

Exhibit 16-4 Drugs That Cause Myalgia

Antihistamines
Antituberculous drugs

drug-induced complaint is one of exclusion of other possibilities and not of primary consideration.

The medications in this chapter are grouped under types of drugs. This list is in no way all encompassing and the reader is referred to more in-depth sources for further information.

Exhibit 16-5 Drugs That Cause Osteoporosis or Fractures

Anticoagulants
Corticosteroids

Antibiotics
- Aminoglycosides (dizziness, vertigo, ataxia)
  Amikacin (Amikin)
  Gentamicin (Garamycin)
  Kanamycin (Kantrex)
  Neomycin
  Streptomycin
  Tobramycin (Nebcin)
- Anti-Fungal Drugs (CNS disturbances)
  Amphotericin B
  Griseofulvin
- Anti-Tuberculous Drugs (myalgia, hyperreflexia)
  Isoniazid
- Anti-viral (dizziness, ataxia)
  Amantadine (Symmetrel)
  Azidothymidine (AZT, Retrovir, Zidovudine)
- Penicillins
  Amoxicillin
  Ampicillin
  Penicillin G
  Oxacillin
- Polypeptides (paresthesias, dizziness, weakness)
  Polymyxin B
- Sulfonamides (headaches, peripheral neuritis, arthritis)
  Sulfamethoxazole (Gantanol)
  with Trimethoprim (Bactrim, Septra)
- Tetracyclines (dizziness, vertigo)
  Minocycline
- Miscellaneous (neurologic disturbances)
  Metranidazole
  Nitrofurantoin (Macrodantin)
  Rifampin (Rifadin)
  Vancomycin (Vancocin)

Anticoagulants
- Heparin (osteoporosis , spontaneous fractures)

Antihistamines
- Histamine H_2 Receptor Antagonists (weakness)
  Diphenhydramine (Benadryl)
- Histamine H_2 Receptor Antagonists (myalgia)
  Cimetidine (Tagamet)
  Famotidine

Antihypertensives
- Beta Blockers (weakness, fatigue)
  Propranolol (Inderal)
  Metoprolol (Lopressor)

Nadolol (Corgard)
- Diuretics (weakness, paresthesia, precipitation of gout)
  Furosemide (Lasix)
  Hydrochlorothiazide
- Vasodialators (headache, fatigue, muscle spasm, peripheral neuropathy)
  Hydralazine
  Nitroprusside
  Prazosin (Minipress)

Central Nervous System Drugs
- Amphetamines (tremors, dizziness)
- Antidepressants (headache, tremors, vertigo, hyperreflexia)
  Amitriptyline (Elavil)
  Doxepin (Sinequan)
  Imipramine (Tofranil)
- Sedatives (headache, ataxia, weakness)
  Diazepam (Valium)
  Lorazepam (Ativan)
  Meprobamate (Equanil)
- Sympatholytics (weakness, fatigue)
  Beta Blockers (Inderal)

Cancer Chemotherapy
- Alkaloids (paresthesia, weakness, loss of DTRs)
  Vinblastine (Velban)
  Vincristine (Oncovin)
- Antimetabolites (cerebellar dysfunction)
  5-flourouracil
- Miscellaneous (CNS dysfunction)
  Asparaginase (Elspar)
  Procarbazine (Matulane)

Coronary Vasodialators
- Calcium Channel Blockers
  Nifedipine (Procardia)
  Verapamil
- Dipyridamole (headache, vertigo)
  Persantine
- Nitrates (headache)
  Isorbide Dinitrate (Sorbitrate)
  Nitroglycerin (sublingual)

Gout
- Colchicine

Nonsteroidal Antiinflammatory Drugs (NSAIDs)
- Indomethacin (headache, dizziness)
  Indocin

- Miscellaneous (CNS symptoms)
  Ibuprofen (Motrin)
  Naproxen (Naprosyn)
  Sulindac (Clinoril)
  Tolmetin (Tolectin)

Steroids
- Glucocorticoids (osteoporosis, fractures, tendon rupture)
  Cortisone
  Dexamethasone (Decadron)
  Hydrocortisone
  Methylprednisolone (Medrol)
  Prednisone
  Prednisolone

BIBLIOGRAPHY

Physician's desk reference. 1989. Oradell, N.J.: Medical Economics Company, Inc.

IV

Management Protocols

17

Sprain/Strain Protocols

INTRODUCTION

Sprain/strain injuries are some of the most common lesions seen in the chiropractic private practice. It is essential that the treating doctor be able to differentiate sprain from strain (Table 17-1), as the protocols may differ somewhat for each, especially when instability is suspected.

After it has been ensured that the patient suffering an acute sprain/strain injury has no fracture, dislocation, or ligamentous instability, treatment may be initiated. The following therapy will provide benefit for the patient. (The mnemonic BRACE is useful in remembering this specific treatment protocol [Exhibit 17-1]).

BANDAGE/BRACE

The use of a brace or bandage will help with both the stability, compression, and restriction of motion in the affected extremity. The brace should not be so tight that it restricts circulation but it should be tight enough

Table 17-1 Differential Diagnosis of Sprain from Strain

Test	Sprain	Strain
Distraction	Pain	Pain
Active motion	Pain	Pain
Isometric (contraction)	No pain	Pain

Exhibit 17-1 Sprain/Strain Mnemonic

> B —Bandage/brace
> R —Rest/rehabilitation
> A—Apply ice
> C—Compression/crutches/chiropractic
> E —Elevation

to allow compression and restriction of motion. Pulses should be taken after brace or bandage application to insure adequate vascular status.

The proper type of brace or bandage depends on the type of injury. Rigid immobilization is used with severe grade II and grade III injuries. Less severe sprain/strain injuries may be treated with an elastic wrap or less rigid forms of immobilization technique. Prolonged immobilization, which can result in adhesive capsulitis, should be avoided if at all possible.

It should be remembered that bracing after an injury is helpful, especially with lesions that are prone to reinjury, such as inversion ankle sprains.

REST/REHABILITATION

Resting injured muscles, ligaments, and tendons is an integral component of therapy. Bear in mind, however, that prolonged inactivity can result in ligament fibrosis, muscle atrophy, and even disuse atrophy of bone. The injured joint should be immobilized for no longer than 7–10 days without the institution of at least some passive range of motion exercises. As pain subsides and the patient regains function, active and resisted ranges of motion with programmed rehabilitation may be begun.

Rehabilitation begins with testing of the involved joint. After the degree of injury, the structures involved, and any specific factors that may have weakened the joint and led to the injury have been established, rehabilitation is begun.

Most often, the goals of rehabilitation can be accomplished and the patient can return to full activity in a relatively short period of time (see Exhibit 17-2). Strengthening weak muscle groups helps add to the

Exhibit 17-2 Goals of Rehabilitation

Restoration of function
Prevention of reinjury
Increase range of motion
Decrease disability

strength and stability of a joint and helps prevent reinjury as well.

APPLY ICE

Cryotherapy has a number of benefits of which vascular constriction, which helps reduce capsular edema and soft tissue swelling, is only one (see Exhibit 17-3). After the injury becomes subacute, a contrast bath (alternating heat and cold) is often helpful.

COMPRESSION

Compression of the involved extremity helps reduce soft tissue swelling and allows passive range of motion exercises to begin more quickly. Compression is accomplished by the application of a bandage as noted above.

CRUTCHES

The proper use of crutches for lower extremity injuries helps rest the joint and provide for appropriate healing. This form of therapy is usually reserved for more severe injuries. If the patient complains that the

Exhibit 17-3 Benefits of Cryotherapy

Decreased capsular swelling
Decreased soft tissue swelling
Control of hemorrhage
Anesthesia

crutches are uncomfortable then they should be raised or lowered for better fit. Improper crutch fitting can result in brachial plexus palsies.

CHIROPRACTIC CARE

The use of manipulation in joint injuries is usually reserved for subacute and chronic disease. This treatment helps to prevent the development of fibrous adhesions within the joint and also helps restore proper joint motion. Adjustment of the affected joint may be performed with caution on an acute injury. Contraindications to manipulation of a joint that has been sprained include fracture, dislocation, or an unstable joint.

ELEVATION

Elevating the involved joint above the level of the heart, if at all possible, facilitates vascular return and helps reduce edema. Elevation should be performed whenever the patient is nonambulatory.

UNSTABLE INJURIES

If there is suspicion that a sprain/strain injury has resulted in an unstable joint, further investigation is warranted. Evaluation for instability begins with plain film radiography, which may be supplemented by stress radiography, arthrography, and/or arthroscopy. These procedures will not only help identify the presence of instability but they will also distinguish which ligament is involved and the severity of the injury. Arthroscopy also has the added benefit of allowing surgical correction of the lesion without necessitating another operation in many cases.

BIBLIOGRAPHY

Beary, J., C. Christian, and T. Sculco, eds. 1981. *Manual of rheumatology and outpatient orthopedic disorders*. Boston: Little, Brown & Co.

Berquist, T. 1986. *Imaging of orthopedic trauma and surgery.* Philadelphia: W.B. Saunders Co.

Rammamurti, C. 1979. *Orthopedics in primary care.* Baltimore: Williams & Wilkins Co.

18

Cervical Spine Trauma Protocols

INTRODUCTION

The patient who presents with acute cervical spine trauma can be enigmatic if not handled properly. Sequelae, from chronic pain to quadriplegia and even death, can occur if the patient is improperly dealt with during examination.

A patient who has sustained trauma to the neck, usually from a motor vehicle accident, is often in a great deal of pain. It is ironic that many times the amount of pain has little to do with the severity of the problem. Many patients have sustained life-threatening injuries in simple "fender bender" accidents where little to no pain was experienced.

EXAMINATION

The first procedure to be performed on a patient with trauma to the neck is to place the patient in a cervical collar. The collar should not be removed until it is verified that the patient does not have any serious injury that may be unstable and result in neurological damage.

The initial examination should include a history of the trauma and a search for any contributory past medical history, such as previous accidents, fractures, or conditions that might predispose the patient to more severe injury from a trauma to the neck.

A brief and concise neurological history and an examination are also of paramount importance. The patient should be questioned as to sensory and motor losses, dizziness, vertigo, visual disturbances, loss of consciousness, and mental status (orientation). There are a number of signs and symptoms that should lead the doctor to believe that serious consequences may follow (Exhibit 18-1).

A brief neurological examination consisting of pupillary examination and response to light, cranial nerve examination, deep tendon reflexes, otoscopic examination (rhinorrhea), and motor and sensory screening examinations should also be performed.

If the patient complains or visceral damage is suggested by the neurological history, the involved areas should also be inspected.

RADIOGRAPHY

The primary study for the investigation of cervical spine trauma is the Davis series (Exhibit 18-2). Some institutions will also include articular pillar views as an ancillary portion of the examination. This view is excellent for demonstration of the articular facets.

The Davis series should be performed within a very specific arrangement, beginning with the neutral lateral cervical projection (remembering that the patient should remain in the cervical collar until at least this view is completed). This film is then developed and screened for any gross pathology, as it is the best projection for depicting unstable injuries. If it is deemed that no instability exists, the collar can be

---

Exhibit 18-1 Signs/Symptoms of Neurologic Sequelae

Severe headache
Visual field loss
Seizure
Blood behind tympanum
Serous otorrhea/rhinorrhea
Loss of consciousness
Sensory losses
Hemiplegia/paraplegia/quadraplegia
Loss of bowel and/or bladder control

Exhibit 18-2 Davis Series

Neutral lateral
AP open mouth
AP lower cervical
Flexion
Extension
Right oblique
Left oblique

removed, if warranted. If not, the remainder of the radiographic examination should be performed in the collar.

The AP open mouth view should be performed and developed next. A search is made for odontoid fractures and burst fracture of C1 in addition to any signs of ligamentous instability. The AP lower cervical, flexion, and extension laterals and obliques complete the study. Pillars views are added if necessary.

If at any time during the examination the doctor feels that neurologic damage is imminent, CT or MRI procedures may be performed. Other ancillary radiographic studies included radionuclide bone scanning, plain film tomography, and myelography.

The protocols outlined above are diagrammed in Figure 18-1. These protocols may vary with each institution. Check with the radiology department chairperson for specific instructions.

After it is confirmed that there are no contraindications to manipulation and the patient can benefit from chiropractic care, treatment can begin.

PHYSICAL THERAPY

Cervical spine adjusting in a patient in acute pain from a whiplash injury is often too painful for the patient to tolerate. In those instances, physical therapy can be very beneficial (Exhibit 18-3). The goals of therapy in this instance are to reduce pain, reduce muscle spasm, and control swelling (both muscular and capsular). These goals can be accomplished with the use of cryotherapy, analgesia with interferential current, and the use of a soft cervical collar. It is understood that a soft cervical collar does not restrict motion

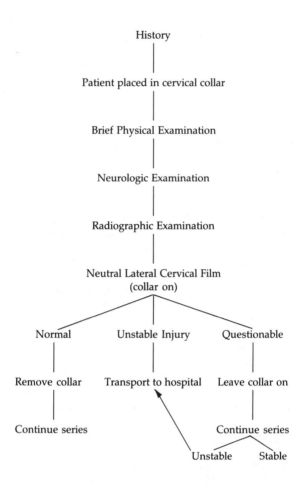

Figure 18-1 Evaluation of the Acute Cervical Spine Trauma Patient

Exhibit 18-3 Physical Therapy for Acute Whiplash Injuries

Ice
Soft cervical collar
Interferential current

but instead functions as a constant reminder to the patient to be aware of the injury.

MANIPULATION

Adjusting the cervical spine after an injury can be accomplished with success but should be performed with caution so as not to aggravate already inflamed tissues. At times, it may be better to begin with light mobilization techniques.

ANCILLARY THERAPIES

Ancillary therapies are summarized in Exhibit 18-4. The use of analgesics such as aspirin, ibuprofen, and acetaminophen can be helpful in cases of moderate to severe pain. Rest is an important part of any therapy after a cervical spine injury; however, passive stretching exercises should begin as soon as it is safe for the patient.

Patient education regarding the side effects of a whiplash injury is also important. After careful scrutiny that no life-threatening sequelae are apparent, the patient should be assured that common side effects following this type of injury (Exhibit 18-5) are troublesome but will dissipate in a short time, in most cases.

Exhibit 18-4 Ancillary Therapy

Analgesia
  Ibuprofen
  Aspirin
  Acetaminophen
Rest
Patient education
  Side effects will subside
  Posture
  Sleeping habits

Exhibit 18-5 Side Effects of Whiplash

Dizziness
Vertigo
Headaches
TMJ pain
Nausea & vomiting
Visual defects
Ataxia
Sleep disturbance

BIBLIOGRAPHY

Bailey, R. 1974. *The cervical spine.* Philadelphia: Lea and Febiger.

Calliet, R. 1977. *Soft tissue pain and disability.* Philadelphia: F.A. Davis.

Daffner, R. 1988. *Imaging of vertebral trauma.* Gaithersburg, Md.: Aspen Publishers, Inc.

Miller, M., J. Gehweiler, and S. Martinez. 1978. Significant new observations on cervical spine. *Am J Roentgenol* 130:659.

Penning, L. 1978. Normal movements of the cervical spine. *Am J Roentgenol* 130:317.

White, A., and M. Panjabi. 1978. Basic kinematics of the human spine; Review of past and current knowledge. *Spine* 3:12.

19

Low Back Pain Protocols

INTRODUCTION

The diagnostic and therapeutic approach to low back pain is, to say the least, fragmented at times. This chapter presents an approach based on a compilation of many different disciplines.

DIAGNOSIS

Investigation of the complaints of a patient with low back pain can be well accomplished if only a simple rule is remembered. In the case of acute pain, it is important to rule out lesions such as fracture and instability first and then concentrate on arriving at the final diagnosis. In other words, are there any contraindications to manipulation of the patient's lumbar spine?

Figure 19-1 will help guide the investigation of the patient presenting with low back pain.

TREATMENT

It is beyond the scope of this book to list all the specific techniques, both manipulative and otherwise, for treating low back pain. Instead, it is felt that the clinical judgment of the doctor will serve as the best indicator of which therapies will most effectively serve the patient's needs.

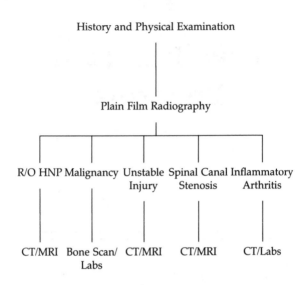

Figure 19-1 Investigation of Low Back Pain

Acute Low Back Pain

While the therapeutic approach to chronic low back pain can take many paths, treatment of acute low back pain is initially directed at reducing pain, decreasing muscle spasm, and reducing soft tissue and capsular swelling so that the patient can return to the normal activities of daily living. The therapy listed below is one suggested approach to the initial treatment of acute low back pain (Exhibit 19-1).

The antigravity position, with the patient prone and the buttocks elevated above the head and feet, is often

---

Exhibit 19-1 Acute Low Back Pain Treatment

Antigravity position
Cryotherapy
Interferential current
Lumbosacral support
Bed rest
Stool softener
Analgesics
TENS unit
Manipulation (if indicated)

times helpful in reducing pain. Cryotherapy, 20 minutes every 2 hours, will help reduce swelling; interferential current can relieve some, if not all, of the pain. A rigid lumbar support, short periods of bedrest with bathroom privileges as needed, a stool softener, and analgesics are helpful therapeutic adjuncts. Transcutaneous electrical nerve stimulation (TENS) can be utilized as well. (While it is understood that use of some of these medications are prohibited by state laws, the therapy can be modified to fit any situation.)

Manipulation of the patient with acute low back pain should be performed with some caution. In selected instances, manipulation can be performed on the first visit but this decision must be made on a case-by-case basis.

Treatment can be performed once daily until there is a significant reduction in pain and return to functional capacity. Treatment should be performed in an intensive care unit or the office until it is deemed that the patient may be released with the home instructions listed above. Thereupon, the treatment schedule should be modified to patient needs.

Chronic Low Back Pain

The treatment of chronic low back pain is usually directed at restoring functional capacity, relieving pain, and eliminating any disability the patient may be suffering.

Pain relief can be accomplished by utilizing standard manipulative techniques and soft tissue therapy, such as massage and passive stretching. Physical therapy modalities, such as interferential current, galvanic current, ultrasound, traction, and heat, can be helpful alone or in combination with each other. It is best to

---

Exhibit 19-2 Chronic Low Back Pain Treatment

Manipulation
Massage
Stretching
Therapeutic exercise
Physical therapy
Lifestyle modification

use what is most comfortable for the patient and what yields the best therapeutic results. (See Exhibit 19-2).

Return to functional capacity and relief of disability can be accomplished in a number of different ways, including passive and active stretching, programmed rehabilitation with therapeutic exercises, and, if necessary, modification of the patient's lifestyle.

BIBLIOGRAPHY

Deyo, R. 1983. Conservative therapy for low back pain. *JAMA* 250:1057.

Deyo, R., A. Diehl, and M. Rosenthal. 1986. How many days of bed rest for acute low back pain? *N Engl J Med* 315:1064.

Hall, H. 1983. Examination of the patient with low back pain. *Bull Rheum Dis* 33:1.

Lawrence, D., ed. 1990. *Fundamentals of chiropractic diagnosis and management.* Baltimore: Williams & Wilkins Co.

Ruge, D., and L. Wiltse. 1977. *Spinal disorders: Diagnosis and treatment.* Philadelphia: Lea and Febiger.

20

Contraindications to Chiropractic Manipulation

Chiropractic manipulation, with all of its beneficial effects (Exhibit 20-1), cannot be performed on all patients. Some of the more common indications for spinal manipulation are listed in Exhibit 20-2. The contraindications listed in this chapter must be considered before adjusting any patient.

There are two categories of contraindications to spinal manipulative therapy. An absolute contraindication is one where, under no circumstances, should high force forms of manipulation be performed on the area of disease until the reason for the contraindication is corrected. This does not imply that low force techniques and/or manipulation in other areas of the spine cannot be performed.

A relative contraindication, on the other hand, is one where certain types of adjustments or the force by which the adjustment is given must be altered to compensate for the problem. Due to the variety of chi-

Exhibit 20-1 Benefits of Manipulation

Pain relief
Restoration of range of motion
Relief of disability
Return to activities of daily living
Muscle strengthening
Improved gait
Improved posture

Exhibit 20-2 Common Indications for Spinal Manipulation

Degenerative joint disease
Disc bulge
Headaches
Herniated nucleus pulposus
Joint pain
Myofascial pain syndromes
Neuralgias
Scoliosis
Sprain/strain
Subluxation

ropractic techniques available today, no attempt will be made to suggest the types of techniques that should be utilized or any modification to any technique.

The lists that follow are not all inclusive and it must be remembered that clinical judgment in each individual case is the best indication or contraindication for chiropractic treatment. In other words, because a condition is listed in this chapter does not by itself mean a patient with that condition should not be manipulated.

ABSOLUTE CONTRAINDICATIONS

Patients with the following problems should not have dynamic high force manipulation in the area(s) of disease.

Entire Spine

- Benign bone tumors (aggressive types)
  Aneurysmal bone cyst
  Giant cell tumor
  Osteoblastoma
  Osteoid osteoma
- Cord tumor
- Dislocation
- Fracture (acute)
- Inflammatory arthritis (acute)
- Infection (osteomyelitis/septic diskitis)

- Instability
- Hematoma (cord or intracanilicular)
- Malignancy
- Meningeal tumor
- Myelopathy (e.g., severe central herniated nucleus pulposus)
- Radiculopathy (with atrophy/severe muscle weakness)

In addition to the above contraindications, which apply to the entire spine, there are a number of conditions that should not be manipulated in each spinal region.

Cervical Spine

- Anomalies (e.g., unstable os odontoideum, dens hypoplasia)
- Arnold-Chiari malformation (upper cervical spine)
- Atlantoaxial instability (upper cervical spine)
- Basilar invagination (upper cervical spine)
- Cerebral ischemic syndromes (e.g., vertebrobasilar artery insufficiency)

Thoracic Spine

- Aortic aneurysm (dissecting type)
- Diastematomyelia

Lumbar Spine

- Abdominal aortic aneurysm (dissecting type)
- Cauda equina syndrome

RELATIVE CONTRAINDICATIONS

This section lists those diseases that mandate that the type and/or force used for manipulation must be altered to prevent serious injury to the patient. In most cases, patients with the following conditions can be safely manipulated but caution must be used.

- Anti-coagulant therapy
- Benign bone tumors (nonaggressive types)
- Fibrous dysplasia
- Hemangioma
- Cerebrovascular accident (history of)
- Clotting/bleeding disorders
- Spinal canal stenosis
- Intervertebral foraminal stenosis
- Fracture (healed injury without instability)
- Lateral recess stenosis
- Osteoporosis
- Pregnancy
- Seizures
- Spondylolisthesis (progressive unstable types)
- Syringomyelia

BIBLIOGRAPHY

Calliet, R. 1981. *Neck and arm pain*. Philadelphia: F.A. Davis.

Calliet, R. 1981. *Low back pain syndrome*. Philadelphia: F.A. Davis.

Lawrence, D., ed. 1990. *Fundamentals of chiropractic diagnosis and management*. Baltimore: Williams & Wilkins Co.

21

Physical Therapy in Chiropractic

INTRODUCTION

The use of physical therapy in the chiropractic practice is commonplace. Such modalities can have a beneficial effect on the clinical outcome of patients in many cases. They must be used judiciously, however, as they are not without side effects and contraindications.

EFFECTS OF PHYSICAL THERAPY MODALITIES

The basic effects of physical therapy modalities can be divided into three categories: thermal, chemical, and kinetic. The type of effect desired is the basis for deciding what therapy to use. Many of the modalities have more than one effect. For example, if the desired effects are a decrease in soft tissue swelling and analgesia, cryotherapy would be helpful in obtaining both. Table 21-1 lists the more commonly used modalities and their primary and secondary effects.

SPECIFIC PHYSICAL THERAPY MODALITIES

This section will outline the use of the various modalities with regard to their indications, contraindications, and physical application.

Table 21-1 Modalities and Their Effects

Modality	Effect
Cryotherapy	Hypothermia
	Decongestion
	Vasoconstriction
	Analgesia
Heat	Hyperthermia
	Vasodilatation
	Analgesia
	Muscle relaxation
Ultrasound	Heating
	Micromassage
Galvanic current	Electrochemical
	Decongestion
Sine current	Muscle contraction
	Decongestion

Cryotherapy

The use of ice has been a treatment for disease for many years. Its effects include vasoconstriction, tissue decongestion, and an anti-inflammatory/analgesic effect. Ice is used most commonly in the treatment of acute diseases to reduce swelling and provide analgesia (Exhibit 21-1). Ice should not be used in patients with a number of different diseases. These are outlined in Exhibit 21-2. Ice should be applied over an area with protection by a towel or wrap of some sort. This helps prevent the onset of frostbite. Typical treatment times vary from 10 to 20 minutes. Home cryotherapy can also be useful if clinically indicated.

A special form of cryotherapy, called ice massage, is used in acute sprain/strain incidents. It is helpful in creating anesthesia after massaging ice over an area for a period of about 5–10 minutes. The patient will expe-

Exhibit 21-1 Indications for Cryotherapy (Acute Diseases)

Sprains
Strains
Bursitis
Arthritis
Tendinitis
Myositis

Exhibit 21-2 Contraindications for Cryotherapy

Advanced cardiovascular disease
Diabetes mellitus
Raynaud's phenomenon
Sensory loss involving cold perception
Vasospastic diseases

rience four separate sensations from an ice massage: cold, burning, aching, and finally anesthesia.

The use of coolant sprays such as fluorimethane have become popular in recent years. These sprays can be used alone or in combination with passive stretching, the so-called "spray and stretch" technique.

Heat Therapy

Heat has a number of useful effects including vasodilatation, increased phagocytosis, relief of muscle spasm, and analgesia. The use of heat is usually confined to subacute and chronic diseases and is most often provided by hydrocollator packs (Exhibit 21-3). Heat should not be applied in patients whose sensation is diminished, as well as in the conditions listed in Exhibit 21-4.

Heat is applied with a towel or wrap between the heat source and the patient to prevent burns. The patient should be questioned periodically as to com-

Exhibit 21-3 Indications for Heat Therapy

Subacute/Chronic
  Sprains
  Strains
  Arthritis
  Tendinitis
  Bursitis
  Myositis
Premanipulation
Premassage
Muscle spasm

Exhibit 21-4 Contraindications for Heat Therapy

```
Acute inflammation
Hemorrhage
Neoplasia
Gravid uterus
Encapsulated swelling (abscess)
Diabetes mellitus
Acute infection
Sensory deficit to heat
```

fort. Treatment times vary from 10 to 20 minutes. Dry heat is usually less beneficial than moist heat.

Specialized forms of therapeutic heat include diathermy, whirlpool bath (where there is also a massaging effect), and infrared therapy. Diathermy provides the deepest tissue heating of the various modalities whereas infrared heat is superficial.

Contrast Bath

The use of alternating heat and cold has the effect of causing vasodilatation and vasoconstriction with all of its concomitant benefits. This modality is best used in the subacute stage of an injury when decongestion of tissues and the influx of blood to the injured area are the main goals of therapy.

Contrast baths should always begin and end with heat and alternate in a cycle for a sustained period of time. For example, treatment with 4 minutes of heat followed by 1 minute of cold for four cycles is then completed with 4 minutes of heat.

The cold bath should be between 50 and 60 degrees and the hot bath between 105 and 110 degrees.

Ultrasound

Applying high frequency sound waves to the body tissues can produce both a micromassage and deep heating, depending upon which type of ultrasound is used. The list of lesions treatable by ultrasound is long but, generally speaking, when lesions are chronic, ultrasound can be used for both massage and heating effects (Exhibit 21-5). The use of this therapy in acute

Exhibit 21-5 Indications for Ultrasound

Acute (pulsed only)
  Sprain/strain
  Bursitis
  Arthritis
Chronic (continuous)
  Sprain/strain
  Bursitis
  Arthritis
  Myalgia/myositis
  Tendinitis

---

injuries is confined to micromassage to reduce swelling. Because ultrasound generates heat by bouncing off internal structures, it should not be used in the diseases listed in Exhibit 21-6.

Ultrasound should be performed either with a conducting gel placed on the skin over the area to be treated or underwater. These techniques are necessary because the crystal inside the ultrasound head will be destroyed if transmission of the sound waves is attempted through air. The sound head should also be constantly moving and it should not be used over bony prominences in order to prevent tissue burning. The intensity of the dosage may be safely varied between 0.5 and 2.5 watts/centimeter^2. Acute condi-

---

Exhibit 21-6 Contraindications for Ultrasound

Hemorrhage
Malignancy
Over the
  Stellate ganglion
  Gonads
  Gravid uterus
  Eye
  Developing epiphyses
  Bony prominences
Infections
Advanced cardiovascular disease
Diabetes mellitus
Sensory deficit to heat

---

tions are usually treated with low intensity (0.5–1.5) and chronic conditions with relatively high intensity (1.5–2.5). The intensity should be increased by .5 if the technique is used underwater. The time of treatment varies from 5 to 15 minutes.

A special form of ultrasound, called phonophoresis, can be used to drive chemicals, usually analgesics, into the affected area.

Galvanic Current

Direct electrical current has chemical and mechanical properties, depending upon the type of current used. Because the modality is polar, ion transfer occurs, which results in acid and alkaline changes in the body tissues. When interrupted current is used, muscle contraction results, thereby providing the mechanical effects.

Galvanic current has a number of different uses, many of which are outlined in Exhibit 21-7. Generally speaking, the positive pad is used when analgesia is necessary and the negative pad is used for the other effects of this treatment. Contraindications include malignancy, loss of sensation, and passage of the current through the brain or heart.

The application of galvanic current includes the use of a wet dispersal pad and a smaller active pad. The current is much greater at the active pad; this is the pad that should be used for iontophoresis, the driving of ions into the affected area. Remember that the same polarity as the ion must be used on the small pad to repel the ions into the body. The machine should be turned off any time changes in settings, including polarity, are made. This will prevent injury to the patient. Treatment times vary from 10 to 20 minutes and the intensity is to patient tolerance.

Exhibit 21-7 Indications for Galvanic Current

Chronic myalgia/myositis
Adhesions
Muscle spasm

Sinusoidal Current

Alternating electrical current is primarily used to stimulate muscle contraction. It is best used on muscles weakened by some disease state although there are other indications, as noted in Exhibit 21-8. Contraindications are listed in Exhibit 21–9.

The use of AC current is facilitated by the use of wet pads and application over the motor points of muscles. It is best not to prolong therapy to the point of dangerous muscle fatigue.

Interferential Current (IFC)

The primary use of this current is for its analgesic effects in acute pain patients.

Traction

Two types of traction are used in the physical rehabilitation of a patient: sustained and intermittent. Sustained traction is best used to splint an area or cause tissue stretching that will result in relaxation. Intermittent traction is used to "pump" an affected area, such as the intervertebral discs in patients with some form of disc disease. Contraindications to traction are listed in Exhibit 21-10.

The application of traction is best accomplished in the cervical spine with 5 percent of the patient's body weight and in lumbar traction with 25 percent of the patient's weight. All attachments should be snug but not too tight and the patient should be positioned so that the maximal effect will be gained.

Exhibit 21-8 Indications for Sine Current

Muscle weakness/atrophy
Muscle spasm
Chronic myalgia/myositis

Exhibit 21-9 Contraindications for Sine Current

Hemorrhage/hematoma
Use through the heart
Abscess
Malignancy
Fracture

Exhibit 21-10 Contraindications for Traction

Acute inflammatory arthritis
Severe muscle spasms
Acute inflammation
HNP (intermittent traction)
Osteomyelitis
Fracture
Malignancy
Osteoporosis
Spinal cord disease
Pregnancy (lumbar spine traction)

Massage

The main therapeutic effect of massage is mechanical, although there may be some reflex visceral changes as well. The physiologic effects of massage include relaxation, adhesion breakdown, edema reduction, and analgesia. There are many different forms of massage, including pétrissage (muscle kneading), effleurage (stroking massage), tapotement (percussion massage), and vibration. The indications

Exhibit 21-11 Indications for Massage

Sprains
Strains
Tendinitis
Myositis/Myalgia
Arthritis
Bursitis
Psychological stress

Exhibit 21-12 Contraindications for Massage

Malignancy
Osteomyelitis
Hemorrhage
Vascular disease (phlebitis)
Skin infection/ulceration
Varicose veins

Table 21-2 Supports and Their Indications

Appliance	Indication
Cervical collar	Whiplash injury
Heel lift	Lower extremity pain
	Spine pain
	Leg length inequality
Lumbosacral belt	HNP
	Sprain/strain
Braces (extremity)	Acute injury
	Prophylaxis

for massage are listed in Exhibit 21-11 and the contraindications in Exhibit 21-12.

Mechanical Supports

The use of orthotics such as braces, shoelifts, lumbosacral supports, and cervical collars is commonplace in the practice of chiropractic. It is well beyond the scope of this text to describe all the types of supports, as there are so many that are used many different ways. Table 21-2 lists some of the more commonly used supports and their indications.

If supports are used, they should, in general, be used for the least amount of time necessary. Prolonged use of a support may lead to muscle atrophy, weakness, and even adhesive capsulitis.

22

Nutrition

INTRODUCTION

Nutrition now plays an increasingly more important role in health care. The use of nutrition in the care of chiropractic patients can be of much benefit. This chapter outlines the more common forms of nutritional therapy and diets used.

GENERAL DIET PLANS

Chiropractic patients present with a myriad of problems, some of which can be helped by a simple modification in diet.

Bland Diet

A bland diet is indicated in patients presenting with gastrointestinal disorders, such as peptic ulcer disease. This type of diet will reduce secretion of gastric juices.

General recommendations include eating three small meals each day with in-between meal snacks. The patient should not skip any meals. Eating slowly and chewing food thoroughly is also beneficial.

Foods that should be avoided include

- Alcohol
- Black pepper

- Breads with high fat content (e.g., pancakes)
- Caffeinated beverages
- Chili powder
- Chocolate products
- Creamed foods/sauces
- Fried foods
- Meats with high fat content (e.g., sausage)

Low Fat Diet

A low fat diet is indicated in patients who have diseases of the liver, gallbladder, pancreas, and heart. It may also be used in patients on a weight loss program, along with a supervised exercise program.

General recommendations for this type of diet include avoiding foods high in fat content and restricting daily fat intake to 40–50 grams.

Foods to avoid include

- Breads with high fat content (e.g., biscuits)
- Cream/creamed foods
- Desserts other than fresh fruit
- Meats with high fat content (e.g., bacon)
- Milk (except skim)
- Nuts
- Snack foods

NUTRITIONAL CARE FOR SELECTED DISEASES

Many diseases will respond more quickly to treatment with the addition of nutritional supplementation. This section describes a number of conditions germane to chiropractic practice and the recommended nutritional support for those conditions.

Bursitis

- Drink 2 or more litres of water per day
- Avoid caffeine and alcohol
- Consume supplements
  —Vitamin B_{12}
  —Vitamin C
  —Omega-3 fatty acids
  —Bioflavonoids

Constipation
- Drink two or more litres of water per day
- Avoid caffeine
- 25–40 grams of fiber per day
- Five raw fruits per day (at least two apples)
- ½ cup oat bran cereal twice per day
- Consume supplements
  —Folic acid
  —Lactobacillus acidophilus

Ecchymosis
- Maintain adequate caloric intake
- Drink at least two litres of water per day
- 1.0–1.2 grams/kilogram body weight protein intake
- Consume supplements
  —Vitamin C
  —Vitamin E
  —Selenium
  —Zinc
  —Bioflavonoids

Gout
- Avoid foods high in purines

Hypoglycemia
- Six small meals per day
- At least one ounce of protein with each meal
- Diet should consist of
  —20–25% protein
  —30–40% fats (polyunsaturated forms)
  —40–45% carbohydrates (complex form)
- Only one glass of milk per day
- Avoid caffeine and alcohol
- High fibre intake
- Consume supplements
  —Calcium
  —Magnesium
  —Chromium
  —Riboflavin

Hypertension*
- High fibre intake (25–40 grams per day)
- Low fat intake (less than 35 grams per day)
- Low cholesterol intake (less than 250 grams per day)
- Low sodium intake (less than 2 grams per day)
- Avoid caffeine and alcohol

- Consume fresh fruits and vegetables
- Consume supplements
  —B complex vitamins
  —Vitamin C
  —Calcium
  —Magnesium
  —Potassium
  —Zinc
  —Omega-3/Omega-6 fatty acids

Hypercholesterolemia/Hypertriglyceridemia

- Low cholesterol intake (less than 300 mg per day)
- Protein intake of .8 grams/kg of body weight
- Diet should include:
  —50–55% carbohydrates
  —25–30% fats (polyunsaturated)
- Consume ½ cup of oat bran twice per day
- Avoid caffeine, alcohol and sweets
- Avoid milk (except skim)
- Increase intake of raw fruits and vegetables
- Consume supplements
  —B complex vitamins
  —Calcium
  —Copper
  —Magnesium
  —Zinc
  —Nicotinic acid
  —Omega-3/Omega-6 fatty acids
  —Garlic
  —Brewer's yeast

Inflammation

- Adequate caloric intake (40–50 kcal × body weight)
- Protein intake of .8–1.2 g/kg body weight
- Drink 8–10 eight oz glasses of water per day
- Consume supplements
  —Vitamin C
  —Vitamin E
  —Zinc
  —Bromelain
  —Proteolytic enzymes
  —Creatine
  —Bioflavonoids

Muscle Weakness

- Drink at least two litres of water per day
- Adequate caloric intake (35–40 kcal/kg)

- Avoid caffeine and alcohol
- Consume supplements
  —Vitamin E
  —Niacin
  —Phosphorus
  —Potassium
  —Kelp

Muscle Cramps

- Drink 2–3 litres of water per day
- Avoid caffeine, alcohol, and carbonated beverages
- Avoid hyperosmotic fluids
- Consume supplements
  —Vitamin E
  —Calcium
  —Magnesium
  —Potassium

Muscle Pain

- Drink two litres of water per day
- Avoid caffeine and alcohol
- Supplements
  —Biotin
  —Pantothenic acid
  —Selenium

Neuropathy

- Drink two litres of water per day
- Avoid all sweets
- Avoid caffeine and alcohol
- Consume supplements
  —Vitamin B_{12}
  —Niacin
  —Pyridoxine
  —Folic acid
  —Thiamine

Peptic Ulcer Disease

- Eat small meals at least every 3 hours
- Avoid the following:
  —Caffeine and alcohol
  —Smoking
  —Chocolate
  —Fried foods
  —Highly seasoned foods
- Limit fluids to 10 oz every hour
- Consume fruit with skin and seeds removed
- Avoid foods with seeds, nuts, and raisins

- May use bland diet if necessary
- Consume supplements
  —Vitamin A
  —Vitamin C
  —Vitamin E
  —Bioflavonoids
  —Zinc sulfate
  —Pyridoxine
  —Glutamine

---

*Care should be taken to consult with the patient's medical doctor concerning the patient's cardiovascular status before prescribing any supplements. Excessive intake of lead and cadmium may actually increase blood pressure.

Appendix A
Abbreviations in Chiropractic

The following is a list of abbreviations and acronyms and their meanings. These will help make medical record keeping much less time consuming and hence more efficient. This list is certainly not all encompassing but should serve as a helpful guide. Entertain the possibility of modifying and adding to this list so that it fits your practice specifically.

ā—ante, "before"

Ⓐ—abnormal

aa—artery, arteries

AAA—abdominal aortic aneurysm

A&O × 4—alert and oriented to person, place, time and situation

Ab—antibody

ABD—abdomen

a.c.—*ante cibum* (before eating)

ACJ—acromioclavicular joint

acid phos—acid phosphatase

ACTH—adrenocorticotrophic hormone

ADH—anti-diuretic hormone

ADL—activities of daily living

ad lib—*ad libitum* (as much as wanted)

AFB—acid-fast bacilli

AFP—alphafeto protein

ag—antigen

A/G—albumin/globulin ratio

AIDS—acquired immunodeficiency syndrome

alk phos—alkaline phosphatase

ALS—amyotrophic lateral sclerosis

ALT—alanine aminotransferase (formerly SGPT)

a.m.—morning

AMA—against medical advice

amb—ambulate

AMPLE—allergies, medications, PMH, LMP, events of illness

ANA—antinuclear antibody

ant—anterior

AP—anteroposterior

APGAR—appearance, pulse, grimace, activity, respirations

ARC—AIDS related complex

AROM—active range of motion

AS—ankylosing spondylitis

ASA—acetylsalicylic acid (aspirin)

ASAP—as soon as possible

ASD—atrial septal defect

ASO—antistreptolysin O

AST—aspartate aminotransferase (formerly SGOT)

ASVD—atherosclerotic vascular disease

AXR—abdomen X-ray

Ⓑ—bilateral

BBB—bundle branch block

BCP—birth control pill

BE—barium enema

b.i.d.—*bis in die* (twice a day)

bili—bilirubin

BM—bowel movement

BMR—basal metabolic rate

BP—blood pressure

BPH—benign prostatic hypertrophy

bpm—beats per minute

BRBPR—bright red blood per rectum (hematochezia)

BRP—bathroom privileges

BS—bowel sounds, breath sounds

BUN—blood urea nitrogen

Bx—biopsy

B9—benign

c̄   —*cum* (with)

C—celcius, centigrade

CA—cancer

Ca—calcium

CABG—coronary artery bypass graft

CAD—coronary artery disease

CADS—cervical acceleration/deceleration syndrome

cap—capsule

CAT—computerized axial tomography

CBC—complete blood count

CC—chief complaint

cc—cubic centimeter

CDA—crystal deposition arthropathy

CF—cystic fibrosis

CHF—congestive heart failure

CI—contraindication

Cl—chloride

cm—centimeter

CMC—carpometacarpal joint

CMT—chiropractic manipulative therapy

CNI-CNXII—cranial nerves one through twelve

CNS—central nervous system

c/o—complaining of

CO—occiput

coc—coccyx

COPD—chronic obstructive pulmonary disease

CP—cerebral palsy

CPK—creatine phosphokinase

  CPBB—brain band

  CPMB—myocardial band

CPMM—muscle band

CPPD—calcium pyrophosphate arthropathy

CPR—cardiopulmonary resuscitation

CRP—C-reactive protein

CSF—cerebrospinal fluid

CT—computerized tomography

CTA—connective tissue arthropathies

CV—cardiovascular

CVA—cerebrovascular accident

CVAT—costovertebral angle tenderness

c/w—consistent with

CXR—chest X-ray

C1-C7—first through seventh cervical vertebrae

DAMA—discharged against medical advice

D&C—dilatation and curretage

d/c—discontinue

DDx—differential diagnosis

diff—differential count (in the CBC)

DIP—distal interphalangeal joint

DISH—diffuse idiopathic skeletal hyperostosis

DJD—degenerative joint disease

DKA—diabetic ketoacidosis

DM—diabetes mellitus

DP—dorsalis pedis (artery)

DPT—diphtheria, pertussis, tetanus

d/t—due to

DTR—deep tendon reflex

DVT—deep vein thrombosis

Dx—diagnosis

Dz—disease

EBV—Epstein-Barr virus

ECG—electrocardiogram

EDC—estimated date of confinement

EEG—electroencephalogram

(E) ENT—(eyes), ears, nose, throat

EKG—electrocardiogram

EMG—electromyogram

EMS—electrical muscle stimulation

EMT—emergency medical technician

EOA—erosive osteoarthritis

EOMI—external ocular muscles intact

EORP—end of range pressure

ER—emergency room

ESR—erythrocyte sedimentation rate

Etiol—etiology

ETOH—ethanol (intoxication)

exac—exacerbation

ext—extension

F—farenheit

FBS—fasting blood sugar

FCNS—fever, chills, night sweats

FD—flexion distraction, fibrous dysplasia

FEV1—forced expiratory volume in one second

FHx—family history

flex—flexion

F→N—finger to nose test

FTA-ABS—fluorescent treponema antibody-absorbed

F/U—follow-up

FUO—fever of unknown origin

Fx—fracture

g—gram

GC—gonorrhea

GGT—gamma-glutamyl transpeptidase

GHJ—glenohumeral joint

GI—gastrointestinal

G/P/A—gravida/para/aborta

GPF—gross physical findings

gr—grain

GSW—gunshot wound

gt., gtt.—*gutta* (drop, drops)

GTT—glucose tolerance test

GU—genitourinary

gyn—gynecologist

h—hour(s)

HA—headache

HADD—hydroxyapatite deposition disease

H&P—history and physical examination

HBP—high blood pressure

HCG—human chorionic gonadotropin

HCO₃—bicarbonate

Hct—hematocrit

HDL—high density lipoprotein

HEENT—head, eyes, ears, nose, throat

Hg—mercury

Hgb—hemoglobin

H/H—hemoglobin/hematocrit

HIV—human immunodeficiency virus (or human T-lympho-cyte virus)

HLA—histocompatibility locus antigen

HNP—herniated nucleus pulposus

H/O—history of

HPI—history of present illness

HR—heart rate

H→S—heel to shin test

h.s.—*hora somni* (hour of sleep—at bedtime)

HSM—hepatosplenomegaly

ht.—height

HTLV-III—human lymphotropic virus-type III

HTN—hypertension

HVG—high volt galvanism

H/W—height/weight

Hx—history

I&O—intake and output

IC—intermittent claudication

ICS—intercostal space

ICU—intensive care unit

IDDM—insulin dependent diabetes mellitus

IFC—interferential current

Ig—immunoglobulin

  IgA—albumin

IgD—beta

IgE—gamma

IgG—alpha-1

IgM—alpha-2

IM—intramuscular (injection)

Incid—incidence

inf—inferior

INH—isoniazid (anti-tuberculous drug)

IPJ—interphalangeal joint

IU—international unit

IV—intravenous

IVC—inferior vena cava

IVP—intravenous pyleogram

IVU—intravenous urogram

JCA—juvenile chronic arthritis

JODM—juvenile onset diabetes mellitus

JVD—jugular venous distension

K+—potassium

Kg—kilogram

KUB—kidneys, ureter, bladder (abdomen X-ray)

kVp—kilovoltage potential

Ⓛ—left

Lab—laboratory

LAE—left atrial enlargement

LAM—laminectomy

LAO—left anterior oblique

LAT—lateral

lat flex—lateral flexion

lb.—pound

LBP—low back pain

LDH—lactate dehydrogenase

LDL—low density lipoprotein

LE—lower extremity

LE prep—lupus erythematosus cell preparation

ll—ligament

LLF—left lateral flexion

LLL—left lower lobe (lung)

LLQ—left lower quadrant (abdomen)

LMNL—lower motor neuron lesion

LMP—last menstrual period

LOC—level of consciousness

LP—lumbar puncture

LPO—left posterior oblique

LR—left rotation

L→R—left to right

L/S—lumbosacral

LUL—left upper lobe

LUQ—left upper quadrant

LVG—low volt galvanism

LVH—left ventricular hypertrophy

L1-L5—first through fifth lumbar vertebrae

Ⓜ—murmur

mA—milliampere

mAs—milliampere seconds

MCH—mean cellular hemoglobin

MCHC—mean cellular hemoglobin concentration

MCL—mid-clavicular line

MCP—metacarpophalangeal joint

MCV—mean cellular volume

meds—medications

mets—metastasis

MFTP—myofascial trigger point

mg—milligrams

MI—myocardial infarction

ml—milliliter

mm—millimeter

MM—multiple myeloma

MMI—maximum medical improvement

MMR—measles, mumps, rubella

mo—month

MRI—magnetic resonance imaging

MS—multiple sclerosis

MTP—metatarsophalangeal joint

MVA—motor vehicle accident

Ⓝ—normal

Na+—sodium

NAD—no apparent distress

NARE—no apparent residual effects

NCV—nerve conduction velocity

neg—negative

neuro—neurological examination

NF—negro female

NIDDM—non-insulin-dependent diabetes mellitus

NKA—no known allergies

NKCIM—no known contraindications to manipulation

NKDA—no known drug allergies

NM—negro male

NMS—neuromusculoskeletal

NPH—neutral protamine Hagedorn (insulin)

n.p.o.—*nil per os* (nothing by mouth)

NSAID—non-steroidal anti-inflammatory drugs

NSR—normal sinus rhythm

N/T—numbness and tingling

N&V—nasuea and vomiting

O₂—oxygen

OA—osteoarthritis

OB/GYN—obstetrician/gynecologist

obl—oblique

OCA—oral contraceptive agent

OCG—oral cholecystogram

o.d.—*oculus dexter* (right eye)

OOB—out of bed

OP—osteopenia, osteoporosis

OPLL—ossification of posterior longitudinal ligament

OR—operating room

orthos—orthopedic tests

o.s.—*oculus sinister* (left eye)

OTC—over the counter (medications)

o.u.—both eyes

oz.—ounce

p̄—post, after

PA—posterior-anterior

PAT—paroxysmal atrial tachycardia

Path—pathogenesis

p.c.—*post cibum* (after meals)

PDR—*Physicians' Desk Reference*

PE—physical examination, pulmonary embolism

PERLA—pupils equal and react to light and accommodation

PFT—pulmonary function tests

pH—hydrogen ion concentration

PID—pelvic inflammatory disease

PIP—proximal interphalangeal joint

p.m.—evening

PMH—past medical history

PMI—point of maximum impulse

PMN—polymorphonuclear leukocyte (neutrophil)

pn—pain

PND—paroxysmal nocturnal dyspnea

PO$_4$—phosphorous

p.o.—*per os* (by mouth)

polys—neutrophils

PON—physical, orthopedic, neurologic examination

post—posterior

PPD—purified protein derivative (TB test)

prn—*pro re nata* (as needed)

PROM—passive range of motion

PSS—progressive systemic sclerosis

PT—physical therapy

Pt—patient

PTA—prior to admission

PTH—parathyroid hormone

PTPW—patient tolerated procedures well

PUD—peptic ulcer disease

PVC—premature ventricular contraction

PVD—peripheral vascular disease

Px—prognosis

q—*quaque* (every)

qAM—every morning

q.d.—every day

q.h.—every hour

q.i.d.—four times a day

q.o.d.—every other day

qPM—every evening

®—right

RA—rheumatoid arthritis

Rad—radiology

RAO—right anterior oblique

RBC—red blood cell count

RDA—recommended daily allowance

RF—rheumatoid factor

RHD—rheumatic heart disease

RIA—radioimmunoassay

RICE—rest, ice, compression, elevation

R→L—right to left

RLF—right lateral flexion

RLL—right lower lobe (lung)

RLQ—right lower quadrant (abdomen)

RML—right middle lobe (lung)

R/O—rule out

ROM—range of motion

ROS—review of systems

rot—rotation

RPO—right posterior oblique

RR—right rotation

RRR—regular rate and rhythm

RTC—return to clinic

RUL—right upper lobe (lung)

RUQ—right upper quadrant (abdomen)

Rx—treatment

š—*sine* (without)

S&A—sugar and acetone

SC—subcutaneous

sec—seconds

SGOT—serum glutamic-oxyloacetic transaminase

SGPT—serum glutamic-pyruvic transaminase

Sgy—surgery

SI—sacroiliac joint

SIDS—sudden infant death syndrome

sig—*signa* (write on label)

SL—spondylolisthesis

SLE—systemic lupus erythematosus

SMAC—sequential multiple analysis chemistry (serum chemistry)

SNSA—seronegative spondyloarthropathies

SOAP—subjective, objective, assessment, plans

SOB—shortness of breath

SP—spinous process

S/P—*status post* (the state after)

SPE—(serum) protein electrophoresis

spondylo—spondylolisthesis

sp/st—sprain/strain

S/S—signs and symptoms

STAT—*statim* (immediately)

STD—sexually transmitted disease

STM—soft tissue manipulation

STS—soft tissue swelling

subQ—subcutaneous

sup—superior

SVC—superior vena cava

Sx—symptom

S1-S5—first through fifth sacral segments

$T_3/T_4/T_7$—abbreviations for thyroid hormone assays

T_3—triiodothyronine

T_4—thyroxine

T.AB.—therapeutic abortion

tab—tablet

TAH—total abdominal hysterectomy

TAHBSO—TAH with bilateral salpingo-oophorectomy

T&A—tonsillectomy and adenoidectomy

T&T—taut and tender

TB—tuberculosis

TBR—total bed rest

tbsp—tablespoon

Temp—temperature

TENS—transcutaneous electrical nerve stimulation

TFT—transverse friction therapy

TGs—triglycerides

THEREX—therapeutic exercise

TIA—transient ischemic attack

TIBC—total iron binding capacity

t.i.d.—*ter in die* (three times a day)

TMJ—temporomandibular joint

TMT—tarsometatarsal joint

TNTC—too numerous to count

TO—telephone orders

TP—trigger point, transverse process

TPRBP—temperature, pulse, respiration, blood pressure

TPT—trigger point therapy

TSH—thyroid stimulating hormone

TURP—transurethral resection of the prostate

tw—twice a week

Tx—treatment

T1-T12—first through twelfth thoracic vertebrae

u—unilateral

UA—uric acid

U/A—urine analysis

ud—*ut dictum* (as directed)

UE—upper extremity

UGI—upper gastrointestinal series

UMNL—upper motor neuron lesion

URI—upper respiratory infection

US—ultrasound

UTI—urinary tract infection

VD—venereal disease

VDRL—Venereal disease research laboratory (syphilis test)

VFI—visual fields intact

VLDL—very low density lipoproteins

VO—voice orders

VS—vital signs

vv—vein(s)

w̄—which

WBC—white blood cell count

w/cm²—watts per square centimeter

WDWN—well-developed, well-nourished

WF—white female

wk—week

WM—white male

WNL—within normal limits

wt.—weight

W/U—work-up

x̄—except

ⓧ—subluxation

XR—X-ray

y/o—years old

yr—year

∅—negative, patient denies
⊖—negative

⊕—positive

Δs—changes

>—greater than

<—less than

⌣ —supine

⌐ —seated

/—per

+/−—plus or minus

i, ii, iii—one, two, three, etc.

Index

A

Abbreviations, 219–232
Abdomen, 41–42
    differential diagnosis, 161–165
    radiology, 100
Abdominal mass, differential diagnosis, 163
Acid phosphatase, 85
Adam's position, 48
Admission note, record keeping, 10
Adrenal calcification, differential diagnosis, 161–162
Adson's test, 48
Alanine aminotransaminase, 86
Albumin, 85
Albumin/globulin ratio, 86
Alkaline phosphatase, 86
Allen's test, 48
Allergy, history, 28–29
Alpha-fetoprotein, 86
Amylase, 86
Anisocoria, differential diagnosis, 168
Ankylosing spondylitis, 134–135, 151
Anterior drawer sign, 48
Antibiotic, causing neuromusculoskeletal side effects, 177
Anticoagulant, causing neuromusculoskeletal side effects, 177
Antihistamine, causing neuromusculoskeletal side effects, 177
Antihypertensive, causing neuromusculoskeletal side effects, 177
Antinuclear antibody, 86
Antistreptolysin-O titre, 86
Apley's test, 48–49
Apparent leg length, 49
Arthritides, 151–153
    classification, 129, 130
    radiology, 98–99
Arthritis. *See also* Specific type
    differential diagnosis, 173
    enteropathy, 136
    gouty, 136

psoriasis, 135
ASAP, 11
Aspartate aminotransferase, 87
Atrophy, 69

B

Babinski reflex, 69
Back pain. *See* Low back pain
Basilar invagination, 153
Battle's sign, 43
Bechterew's test, 49
Bicarbonate, 87
Bilirubin, 87
Bladder cancer, 143
Bland diet, 213–214
Block vertebra, 153
Blood smear with Wright's stain, 80–81
Blood specimen tube, 113
Blood urea nitrogen, 87
Bone
   aggressive lesions, 105
   benign lesions, 104
   unstable lesions, 106
Bone cancer, 144
   radiology, 97–98
Bone radiology, 97–98
Bowstring sign, 49
Braggard's test, 49
Brain cancer, 143–144
Brain lesion, 71
   supratentorial vs. infratentorial, 71
Brain stem lesion, 73, 74
Breast cancer, 144
   screening examination, 142–143
Breast examination, 122–123
Brucellosis, 154
Brudzinski's sign, 50
Bursitis, nutrition, 214

C

C-reactive protein, 92
Calcium, 87
Calcium pyrophosphate crystal deposition disease, 136–137
Cancer, 141–149. *See also* Specific type
   clinical examination, 143–146
   diagnostic imaging, 148–149
   laboratory tests, 146–147
   screening examination, 141–143
   spine pain, 155
Cancer chemotherapy, causing neuromusculoskeletal side
   effects, 178
Cardiac murmur, 39, 40

Cardiopulmonary resuscitation, 123–125
Carotid artery testing, 116–117
Case presentation, 22
Central nervous system drug, causing neuromusculoskeletal
    side effects, 178
Cerebellar challenge, 77
Cerebral lesion, 73, 74
Cervical spine
    distraction test, 50
    manipulation contraindications, 201
    spine pain, referred pain, 156–157
Cervical spine trauma protocol, 189–194
    ancillary therapies, 193
    evaluation, 191, 192
    examination, 189–190
    manipulation, 193
    physical therapy, 191–193
    radiography, 190–191
Chart, 5–10. *See also* Record keeping
    blank space, 5
    illegible, 6
Chest
    differential diagnosis, 165–168
    radiology, 100–101
Cheyne-Stokes respiration, 38
Chief complaint, 28
    mnemonic OPPQRST, 28
Chiropractic radiologist, 95
Chloride, 87
Cholesterol, 87
Chvostek's sign, 43
Clinic and ward round, 22
Clinical oncology, 141–149
Clubbing, 43
Coccidioidomycosis, 154
Codman's sign, 50
Colon cancer, 145
    screening examination, 142
Communication, 3–4
Complete blood count, 79–83
    interpretation, 82
    normal values, 80
Compliance, 4
Computerized tomography, 109
    indications, 109
Congenital dysplasia, 153
Congenital lesion, radiology, 100
Constipation, nutrition, 215
Contrast bath, 206
Coolant spray, 205
Coronary vasodilator, causing neuromusculoskeletal side
    effects, 178
Costoclavicular test, 50

Cozen's test, 50
Cranial nerve examination, 76
Creatine phosphokinase, 88
Creatinine, 88
Cryotherapy, 204–205
    contraindications, 205
    effects, 204
    indications, 204
Cullen's sign, 43

D

Decision-making process, 4
Deep tendon reflex, 68, 69
Degenerative joint disease, 137–138, 151
Dejerine's triad, 50
Dementia, differential diagnosis, 169
Dermatome, 69, 70
Diagnostic imaging, 95–111
    advanced, 109–111
Diagnostic ultrasound, 110
    indications, 111
Diet, 213–218
Differential diagnosis
    abdominal mass, 163
    adrenal calcification, 161–162
    anisocoria, 168
    arthritis, 173
    dementia, 169
    dizziness, 169
    dysphagia, 162
    extrapleural sign, 165
    headache, 169
    hematemesis, 162
    hematochezia, 162–163
    hemianopia, 168–169
    hepatomegaly, 163
    hilar enlargement, 165
    hyperreflexia, 169–170
    hyporeflexia, 170
    mediastinal mass, 166–167
    melena, 163
    muscular weakness, 172
    ophthalmoplegia, 170
    pain, 173–174
    pancreatic calcification, 164
    pleural space fluid, 165
    pneumonia, 168
    pneumoperitoneum, 164
    polyneuropathy, 171
    pulmonary nodule, 167, 168
    pulmonary parenchyma consolidation, 165
    renal calcification, 164
    scoliosis, 174

splenic calcification, 164
splenomegaly, 165
syncope, 171–172
tremor, 172
vas deferens calcification, 165
vertigo, 172
Diffuse idiopathic skeletal hyperostosis, 138, 152
Disc bulge, 155
Discharge note, record keeping, 10
Diskitis, 152
Dislocation, 155
Distraction test, cervical spine, 50
Dizziness
differential diagnosis, 169
drugs causing, 176
Doctor-patient relationship, 3–4
Dugas' test, 51
Dysphagia, differential diagnosis, 162

E

Ears, 35–36
Ecchymosis, nutrition, 215
Electrocardiogram, 118–119
Ely's heel-to-buttock test, 51
Enteropathic arthritis, 136, 152
Erythrocyte sedimentation rate, 91
Escherichia coli, 154
Extrapleural sign, differential diagnosis, 165
Extremities, physical examination, 42–43
Eyes, 34–35

F

Face, 33
Facet syndrome, 155
Family history, 29, 30
Fasciculation, 68
Fibrillation, 68
Fibromyalgia syndrome, 138–139
Fibrous dysplasia, 154
Figure four test, 55
Finklestein's test, 51
Fluorescent treponemal antibody, 88
Fracture, 155
drugs causing, 176

G

Gaenslen's test, 51
Galvanic current, 208
effects, 204
indications, 208
Gamma-glutamyl transpeptidase, 88

Genital cancer, 145
    screening examination, 143
Globulin, 88
Glucose, 88
Goldthwait's test, 51
Gout
    causing neuromusculoskeletal side effects, 178
    nutrition, 215
Gouty arthritis, 136

H

Head, 33
Headache
    differential diagnosis, 169
    drugs causing, 175
    evaluation, 170
Heart, 38–41
Heat, effects, 204
Heat therapy, 205–206
    contraindications, 206
    indications, 205
Hematemesis, differential diagnosis, 162
Hematochezia, differential diagnosis, 162–163
Hematocrit, 83
    interpretation, 83
Hemianopia, differential diagnosis, 168–169
Hemoccult, 92
Hemoglobin, 82–83
    interpretation, 82, 82–83
Hepatomegaly, differential diagnosis, 163
Hibbs' test, 52
Hilar enlargement, differential diagnosis, 166
History, 27–31
    allergy, 28–29
    medication, 29
    mnemonic AMPLE, 28–31
    past medical, 29–31
    scoliosis, 59
Homans' sign, 43, 52
Hospital protocol, 21–23
    case presentation, 22
    clinic and ward round, 22
    record keeping, 22
    surgery, 22–23
Human chorionic gonadotropin, 88
Human immunodeficiency virus, 88
Human T-lymphocyte virus, 88
Hydroxyapatite deposition disease, 137
Hypercholesterolemia, nutrition, 216
Hyperparathyroidism, 154
Hyperreflexia, differential diagnosis, 169–170
Hypertension, nutrition, 215–216
Hypertriglyceridemia, nutrition, 216

Hypoglycemia, nutrition, 215
Hyporeflexia, differential diagnosis, 170

I

Ice, 204–205
Iliac compression, 52
Infection, radiology, 99–100
Inflammation, nutrition, 216
Informed consent, record keeping, 10
Interferential current, 209
Interpretation, radiology, 97–101
Intervertebral hypermobility, 153
Intervertebral hypomobility, 153
Iron, 88
Iron binding capacity, 89

J

Jackson's compression test, 52

K

Kemp's test, 52
Kernig's sign, 53
Kidney cancer, 145

L

Laboratory diagnosis, 79–93
Laboratory panel, 92–93
Laboratory profile, 92
Lactate dehydrogenase, 89
Lasègue's test, 53
Leg length, apparent, 49
Lesion, causes, 107
Leukemia, 146
Levine's sign, 44
Lewin's test, 53
Lindner's sign, 53
Lipase, 89
Liver cancer, 145
Low back pain, 195–198
    acute, 196–197
    chronic, 197–198
    diagnosis, 195, 196
    treatment, 195–198
Low fat diet, 241
Lower body screening examination, 65–66
Lumbar spine
    manipulation contraindications, 201
    spine pain, 158
Lumbosacral transitional segment, 153
Lung cancer, 144
    screening examination, 142

Lupus erythematosus cell preparation, 89
Lymphoma, 146

M

Magnetic resonance imaging, 110
    indications, 110
Manipulation
    benefits, 199
    contraindications, 199–202
        absolute, 200–201
        relative, 201–202
    indications, 200
Massage, 210–211
    contraindications, 211
    indications, 210
Maximum cervical compression test, 53
McBurney's sign, 44
McMurray's test, 54
Mean corpuscular hemoglobin, interpretation, 82
Mechanical support, 211
Mediastinal mass, differential diagnosis, 166–167
Medication
    causing neuromusculoskeletal side effects, 175–179
    history, 29
Medication orders, 13–15
Melena, differential diagnosis, 163
Menstrual period, last, 31
Mental status examination, 76
Milgram's test, 54
Mill's test, 54
Minor's sign, 54
Monospot, 89
Motor examination, 76
Motor neuron lesion, upper vs. lower, 68
Murphy's punch test, 44
Murphy's sign, 44
Muscle cramp, nutrition, 217
Muscle pain, nutrition, 217
Muscle weakness
    differential diagnosis, 172
    nutrition, 216–217
Myalgia, drugs causing, 176
Myofascitis, 153

N

Neri's bowing test, 54
Nerve root lesion, 72, 73
Nervous system, differential diagnosis, 168–172
Neurologic examination, screening, 76–77
Neurologic lesion, 67–77
    etiology, 71–74
    location, 67–71

treatment, 74–75
    contraindications, 74–75
Neurological/neurosurgical consultation, 75
Neuropathy, nutrition, 217
Nonsteroidal antiinflammatory drug, causing
   neuromusculoskeletal side effects, 178
Nose, 36
Nucleus pulposus, herniated, 155
Nutrition, 213–218
  bursitis, 214
  constipation, 215
  ecchymosis, 215
  gout, 215
  hypercholesterolemia, 216
  hypertension, 215–216
  hypertriglyceridemia, 216
  hypoglycemia, 215
  inflammation, 216
  muscle cramp, 217
  muscle pain, 217
  muscle weakness, 216–217
  neuropathy, 217
  peptic ulcer disease, 217–218

O

Ober's test, 54–55
Obturator sign, 44
Occipitocervical transitional segment, 153
Oncology, 141–149
  clinical examination, 143–146
  diagnostic imaging, 148–149
  laboratory tests, 146–147
Operative note, record keeping, 10
Ophthalmoplegia, differential diagnosis, 170
Orders
  mnemonic LATER DUDES, 12
  type, 12–13. *See also* Specific type
  writing, 11–15
Orthopedic test, 47–66. *See also* Specific type
  pertinent negative, 47
Orthopedics, 47–66
Orthotics, 211
Ortolani's click test, 55
Osteoarthritis of facet articulations, 152
Osteoporosis, 154
  drugs causing, 176

P

Paget's disease, 154
Pain, differential diagnosis, 173–174
Pancreatic calcification, differential diagnosis, 164
Pancreatic carcinoma, 145

Paralysis, 68
Parathyroid hormone, 89
Paresis, 68
Patrick Fabere test, 55
Peptic ulcer disease, nutrition, 217–218
Peripheral nerve entrapment site, 171
Peripheral nerve lesion, 72
Phlebotomy, 113–116
Phosphorus, 89
Physical examination, 31–44
   scoliosis, 59–60
Physical therapy, 203–212
   effects, 203
Platelet, 83
   interpretation, 83
Pleural space fluid, differential diagnosis, 165
Pneumonia, differential diagnosis, 168
Pneumoperitoneum, differential diagnosis, 164
Polyneuropathy, differential diagnosis, 171
Potassium, 89–90
Prescription
   components, 14–15
   form, 14
   writing, 13–15
Problem–oriented medical record system, 6–10
   comprehensive data base, 6–7
   initial plans, 7, 8–9
   problem list, 8
   progress notes, 8, 9–10
Protein, 90
Protein electrophoresis, 90
Pseudomonas, 154
Psoas sign, 44
Psoriatic arthritis, 135, 152
Pulmonary nodule, differential diagnosis, 167, 168
Pulmonary parenchyma consolidation, differential diagnosis, 165

R

Racoon eyes, 44
Radiation physics, 101–105
Radiculopathy, 72, 73
Radiology, 91–111, 119–121
   abdomen, 100
   arthritides, 98–99
   basic rules, 95–97
   bone tumor, 97–98
   cervical spine trauma protocol, 190–191
   chest, 100–101
   congenital lesion, 100
   differential diagnosis, 101, 102–103
   follow-up imaging, 101, 102–103
   infection, 99–100
   reports, 105–109

rheumatology, 133
    scoliosis, 60–61
    trauma, 99
Radionuclide bone scanning, 110
    indications, 111
Range of motion test, 57–59
Record keeping, 5–10. *See also* Chart
    admission note, 10
    discharge note, 10
    hospital protocol, 22
    informed consent, 10
    operative note, 10
    state statutes, 5
Rectal examination, 121–122
Red blood cell count, 82
    interpretation, 82
Referral, 17–20
    incoming, 19–20
    indications, 17–18
    outgoing, 18–19
    personalized list, 20
    types, 18–20
Reiter's syndrome, 135–136, 152
Renal calcification, differential diagnosis, 164
Renal carcinoma, 145
Review of systems, 29, 30
Rheumatoid arthritis, 134, 153
Rheumatoid factor, 90
Rheumatology, 129–139
    disease classification, 129, 130
    history, 129–131
    laboratory tests, 132–133
    physical examination, 131–132
    radiology, 133
Risser's sign, skeletal maturation, 60–62
Rust's sign, 44

S

Scoliosis
    Cobb measurement method, 60
    differential diagnosis, 174
    evaluation, 59–62
    history, 59
    physical examination, 59–60
    radiology, 60–61
    Risser-Ferguson measurement method, 61
    treatment, 61–62
Screening examination, 64–66
    breast cancer, 142–143
    colon cancer, 142
    genital cancer, 143
    lung cancer, 142
    neurologic, 76–77

Sensory examination, 76
Serum chemistry, 85–91
Serum glutamic-oxaloacetic transaminase, 91
Serum glutamic-pyruvic transaminase, 91
Shoulder depression test, 55
Signature, 6, 12
Sine current, 209
   contraindications, 210
   effects, 204
   indications, 209
Skeletal maturation, Risser's sign, 60–62
Skeleton, differential diagnosis, 173–174
Skin, 33
Sodium, 91
Soto-Hall test, 55
Spinal cord lesion, 69–71, 73, 74, 144
Spine pain, 151–158
   cancer, 155
   cervical spine, referred pain, 156–157
   chiropractic, 153
   developmental, 153
   infectious causes, 154
   lumbar spine, 158
   metabolic causes, 154
   thoracic spine, referred pain, 157–158
   trauma, 155
   vertebrogenic, 151–158
Spinous percussion, 55
Splenic calcification, differential diagnosis, 164
Splenomegaly, differential diagnosis, 165
Splinter hemorrhage, 44
Spondylolisthesis, 62–64, 154
   diagnosis, 63
   pathogenesis, 62–63
   treatment, 63–64
   types, 62–63
Sprain, 154
Sprain protocol, 183–186
   bandage/brace, 183–184
   chiropractic care, 186
   compression, 185
   crutches, 185–186
   differential diagnosis, 183
   elevation, 186
   ice, 185
   mnemonic, 184
   rest/rehabilitation, 184–185
   unstable injuries, 186
Spurling's maneuver, 56
Standing orders, 11
STAT, 11
Sterile technique, 22–23
Steroid, causing neuromusculoskeletal side effects, 179

Stomach cancer, 146
Straight leg raising, 53
Strain, 154
Strain protocol, 183–186
    bandage/brace, 183–184
    chiropractic care, 186
    compression, 185
    crutches, 185–186
    differential diagnosis, 183
    elevation, 186
    ice, 185
    mnemonic, 184
    rest/rehabilitation, 184–185
    unstable injuries, 186
Subluxation, 153
Surgery, 22–23
Syncope, differential diagnosis, 171–172
Synovitis, 155

T

Telephone orders, 11
Thomas test, 56
Thompson's test, 56
Thoracic spine
    manipulation contraindications, 201
    spine pain, referred pain, 157–158
Thorax, 37–38
Throat, 36–37
Thyroid stimulating hormone, 91
Thyroxine, 91
Traction, 209–210
    contraindications, 210
    intermittent, 209
    sustained, 209
Trauma, radiology, 99
Tremor, differential diagnosis, 172
Trendelenburg's test, 56
Triglyceride, 91
Triiodothyronine, 91
Tripod sign, 56
Tuberculosis, 154

U

Ultrasound, 206–208
    contraindications, 207
    effects, 204
    indications, 207
Upper body screening examination, 64–65
Uric acid, 91
Urinalysis, 83–85
    normal, 83
Urine, specimen collection, 116

V

Valgus stress, 57
Valsalva maneuver, 57
Varus stress, 57
Vas deferens calcification, differential diagnosis, 165
Veneral disease research laboratory, 91
Venipuncture, 113–116
Verbal orders, 11
Vertebral anomaly, 153
Vertebrobasilar artery testing, 116–117
Vertebrogenic spine pain, 151–158
Vertigo
    differential diagnosis, 172
    drugs causing, 176
Vital signs, 32–33

W

Weakness, drugs causing, 176
Whiplash
    physical therapy, 191–193
    side effects, 193, 194
White blood cell count, 82
    interpretation, 82
Wright's hyperabduction test, 57
Written orders, 11

Y

Yeoman's test, 57
Yergason's test, 57